W9-BNR-637

Contemporary Guide to Contraception™

Steven T. Nakajima, MD
Associate Professor and Division Chief,
Division of Reproductive Endocrinology
and Infertility
Department of Obstetrics, Gynecology,
and Women's Health
University of Louisville School of Medicine
Louisville, Kentucky

Third Edition

Lake Superior College Library

Published by Handbooks in Health Care Co.,
Newtown, Pennsylvania, USA

This book has been prepared and is presented as a service to the medical community. The information provided reflects the knowledge, experience, and personal opinions of the author, Steven T. Nakajima, MD, Associate Professor and Division Chief, Division of Reproductive Endocrinology and Infertility, Department of Obstetrics, Gynecology, and Women's Health, University of Louisville School of Medicine, Louisville, Kentucky.

This book is not intended to replace or to be used as a substitute for the complete prescribing information prepared by each manufacturer for each drug. Because of possible variations in drug indications, in dosage information, in newly described toxicities, in drug/drug interactions, and in other items of importance, reference to such complete prescribing information is definitely recommended before any of the drugs discussed are used or prescribed.

Photography by Ross Photographics, Inc.

International Standard Book Number: 978-1-931981-76-7

Library of Congress Catalog Card Number: 2007922883

Contemporary Guide to Contraception™.
Copyright© 2007, 2006, 2005 by Handbooks in Health Care Co., a Division of AMM Co., Inc. All rights reserved. Printed in the United States of America. No part of this book may be used or reproduced in any manner whatsoever, including but not limited to electronic or mechanical means such as photocopying, recording, or using any information storage or retrieval system, without written permission, except in the case of brief quotations embodied in critical articles and reviews. For information, write Handbooks in Health Care, 3 Terry Drive, Suite 201, Newtown, Pennsylvania 18940, (215) 860-9600.

Web site: www.HHCbooks.com

Table of Contents

Preface

The goals of this handbook are twofold: (1) to provide a general overview of the subject of contraception, and (2) to be a handy, practical reference source for the health-care provider. The increased use of generic medication has made the task of identifying a patient's contraceptive product more difficult. Therefore, a major focus of the handbook is a color atlas of contraceptive products, which is designed to help the clinician accurately identify a patient's oral contraceptive medication, whether brand name or generic. To further assist clinicians in keeping up with the changing nature of medicine and the field of contraception, each chapter has been supplemented with specific Web sites.

The information in this handbook is not intended to replace the traditional discussion between the health-care provider and the patient, but rather to provide additional information on contraceptive options and to supplement dialogue on different methods. The handbook should not be used to guide therapy; only the health-care provider can decide which treatment plan is appropriate for a given patient. However, it is meant to extend the use of products or methods to help make contraception more convenient and effective.

This handbook contains information on the use of medication for off-label indications. These sections are intended to extend or modify techniques for which there is a reasonable rationale. Clinicians should carefully consider these modifications when using medication for an off-label indication. The author and the publisher are not responsible for omissions, errors, or a change in therapy that arise from new research findings.

Steven T. Nakajima, MD
Louisville, Kentucky

Acknowledgments

The author would like to thank the following individuals for their help in developing and producing this handbook.

Molly Hall: Technical support

Carole Himmelstein, Yama, Inc.: Lea's Shield® sample

Art Jacob, Art Jacob Prescription Shoppe: Oral contraceptive pills

Sherri Luba, CooperSurgical, Inc.: Milex Wide-Seal® Silicone Diaphragm photograph

Anna Manno, Barr Pharmaceuticals, Inc.: Barr OCP samples

Carrie Nakajima: Proofreading and editorial assistance

George Roberts, Pfizer Pharmaceuticals, Inc.: Demulen® OCP sample

Alfred Shihata, FemCap, Inc.: FemCap™ sample

Hillary Steele, Watson Pharmaceuticals, Inc.: Watson OCP samples

Liz Summerhayes, Cervical Cap Ltd.: Prentif™ Cavity-Rim Cervical Cap sample

Mark Szymanski, Ortho-McNeil Women's Health Care: Selected OCP photographs

Beverly Williams: Reference and technical support

Dedication

This handbook is dedicated to my wife, Carrie, and our two daughters, Wendy and Jessica. Thank you for your support in developing this handbook.

Glossary

Common Abbreviations

ACOG:	American College of Obstetricians and Gynecologists
ARHP:	Association of Reproductive Health Professionals
AWP:	average wholesale price
BMD:	bone mineral density
BTB:	breakthrough bleeding
CDC:	Centers for Disease Control and Prevention
CDER:	Center of Drug Evaluation and Research
CI:	confidence interval
CIS:	carcinoma in situ
CREST:	Collaborative Review of Sterilization
DMPA:	depot-medroxyprogesterone acetate
DRSP:	drospirenone
DSG:	desogestrel
DVT:	deep vein thrombosis
EC:	emergency contraception
EE:	ethinyl estradiol
ETD:	ethynodiol diacetate
FAMs:	fertility awareness methods
FDA:	US Food and Drug Administration
IM:	intramuscularly
HIV:	human immunodeficiency virus
HSG:	hysterosalpingogram
ICSI:	intracytoplasmic sperm injection
IUD:	intrauterine device
IUS:	intrauterine system

LNG: levonorgestrel
MI: myocardial infarction
N-9: nonoxynol-9
NET: norethindrone
NETA: norethindrone acetate
NGM: norgestimate
NSFG: National Survey of Family Growth
OCP: oral contraceptive pill
OR: odds ratio
PE: pulmonary embolism
PET: polyethylene terephthalate
PID: pelvic inflammatory disease
PGI_2: prostaglandin I_2
RR: relative risk
STD: sexually transmitted disease
t-PA: tissue plasminogen activator
TXA_2: thromboxane A_2
VTE: venous thromboembolism
WHO: World Health Organization

Chapter 1

Contraceptive Options

There are many different methods that individuals and/or couples can use to prevent conception. The decision to use a particular contraceptive method will often depend on availability, any prior knowledge or experience with the method, the individual's education level or financial status, and the individual's current social situation. However, almost any contraceptive method can be effective, and the use of any method is often less expensive and poses less risk for morbidity and mortality than an unintended pregnancy.[1]

Contraceptive methods can be subdivided into different categories, such as female vs male contraceptives or reversible vs permanent sterilization methods. These distinctions have become less important because it is becoming more common to use a barrier technique (eg, a male condom) in addition to oral contraceptive pills (OCPs) or other contraceptive measures to prevent sexually transmitted diseases (STDs). The practice of combined or 'dual methods' has undoubtedly improved contraceptive efficacy.

Scope of the Problem: Unintended Pregnancies

According to information published by the Alan Guttmacher Institute in February 2004, there are approximately 60 million women in the United States in their childbearing years (15 to 44 years).[2] Approximately 64% of these women (38.4 million) use a contraceptive method, while only 5% of women (3 million) use no method of contraception.

Table 1-1: Comparison of 15 Methods of Contraception

Method	Failure Rate (%)	First-Year Costs* ($)	Five-Year Costs* ($)
Tubal ligation**	0.17	2,554	2,584
Vasectomy**	0.04	763	764
Oral contraceptives	3.00	422	1,784
Progestin implant**	0.32	804	850
Progestin injectable	0.30	285	1,290
Progesterone-T IUD	2.00	449	2,042
Copper-T IUD**	0.42	498	540

Progesterone-T IUD=Progestasert® intrauterine device changed every 12 months
*Costs are for a private payer (managed payment model).
**Failure rates for these methods represent the average of years 1 through 5:
Tubal ligation: 0.4000%, 0.1333%, 0.1333%, 0.1333%, 0.0667%

Each year, there are approximately 3 million unintended pregnancies in the United States. Of these, 47% are in the 3 million women who practice no contraceptive method, and 53% are in women who are using a contraceptive method. Most unintended pregnancies among contraceptive users result from inconsistent or incorrect use of their contraceptive method. Of the approximately 3 million unintended

Method	Failure Rate (%)	First-Year Costs* ($)	Five-Year Costs* ($)
Diaphragm	18.00	852	3,666
Male condom	12.00	533	2,424
Female condom	21.00	1,072	4,872
Sponge***	30.00	1,264	5,700
Spermicides	21.00	913	4,102
Cervical cap***	30.00	1,310	5,730
Withdrawal	19.00	721	3,278
Periodic abstinence†	20.00	759	3,450
No method†	85.00	3,225	14,663

Vasectomy: 0.15%, 0.01%, 0.01%, 0.01%, 0.01%
Progestin implant: 0.09%, 0.31%, 0.40%, 0.40%, 0.40%
Copper-T IUD: 0.8%, 0.2%, 0.6%, 0.2%, 0.3%
***Weighted averages of rates for parous and nulliparous women of reproductive age at risk of pregnancy.
Modified from Trussell et al[1]
†Costs related to unintended pregnancies.

pregnancies, 43% are aborted, 13% end in miscarriage, and 44% result in a live delivery.

Keeping Contraception Methods in Perspective

Although there are risks and complications with any contraceptive method, they should be kept in perspective.

In 1999, pregnancy-related mortality in the United States was 13.2 deaths/100,000 live births.[3] The risk of a pregnancy-related death often far outweighs the risk of any contraceptive approach.

The use of any contraceptive technique, however basic, decreases the chance of conception and is less expensive than pregnancy and birth. In a 1995 study, Trussell et al[1] modeled the direct medical costs of 15 contraceptive methods and examined the 5-year costs and number of pregnancies avoided with each compared with no contraceptive method (Table 1-1). Direct medical costs included the treatment of side effects and unintended pregnancies. For each method, variable percentages of the pregnancies were assumed to end as induced abortions, spontaneous abortions, ectopic pregnancies, or term deliveries. The researchers concluded that if no contraceptive method was used over a 5-year period, 4.25 unintended pregnancies/woman would occur, at a cost of $14,663 each to a private payer. This is called the managed payment model. Trussell and colleagues demonstrated that the use of simple procedures such as periodic abstinence, coital withdrawal, or application of spermicide was effective in decreasing the incidence of pregnancy and saved health-care resources by preventing unintended pregnancies. Over a 5-year period, the copper-T intrauterine device (IUD) and vasectomy were the most cost-effective methods. OCPs, the most commonly used contraceptive method in the United States, had low initial monthly costs, but cumulative costs exceed those of the copper-T IUD after 1 year of use.

In 2003, this research group updated its 1995 report and reviewed the overall cost of nine contraceptive methods available to US women who plan to use contraception for 5 years: the cervical cap, the copper-T IUD, the diaphragm, the female condom, the levonorgestrel-releasing IUD, OCPs, the progestin injectable, spermicide, and tubal ligation.[4] The study did not include the progestin

Table 1-2: Contraceptive Methods of Women in the United States Aged 15-44 Years*

Method	Percent Distribution (±SE)
Oral contraceptive pill	30.6 (0.9)
Female sterilization	27 (0.9)
Male condom	18 (0.7)
Male sterilization	9.2 (0.6)
Progestin injectable	5.3 (0.5)
Withdrawal	4 (0.4)
Intrauterine device	2 (0.3)
Progestin implant, Lunelle™, or patch	1.2 (0.2)
Periodic abstinence—calendar rhythm	1.2 (0.2)
Other methods**	0.9 (0.2)
Periodic abstinence—natural family planning	0.4 (0.1)
Diaphragm	0.3 (0.1)

SE=standard error
*Based on the 2002 National Survey of Family Growth
**Includes Today® Sponge, cervical cap, female condom, and other methods
Modified from Mosher et al[5]

implant and the contraceptive patch or ring. Aside from vasectomy, a method that women do not have direct control over, tubal ligation, the levonorgestrel-releasing IUD, and the copper-T IUD were the most effective methods.

The least expensive methods, accounting for all costs (initial cost, method failure, method discontinuation, and transition to an alternative method), were the levonorgestrel-releasing IUD, the copper-T IUD, and the progestin injectable. Although a tubal ligation is more effective, the higher initial cost may not justify the small increase in contraceptive efficacy. The levonorgestrel-releasing and copper-T IUDs were more cost-effective if a woman was planning for 5 years of contraception. Often, the task is to determine whether a patient will actually use an IUD for 5 years and thus distribute its relatively high initial cost over that period.

Current Use of Contraceptive Methods in the United States

Based on the 2002 National Survey of Family Growth, conducted by the National Center for Health Statistics, the leading method of contraception in the United States in 2002 was the OCP, followed by female sterilization, male condom use, male sterilization, and injectable progestin (Table 1-2).[5] Together, these five methods account for approximately 90% of all methods used by women and men in the United States.

The choice of a contraceptive method can be strongly influenced by the user's level of education,[5] ethnic background, financial status, and social situation.[1] College-educated women are four times as likely to use OCPs, four times as likely to rely on a partner's vasectomy, and one fourth as likely to use female sterilization as their method of contraception compared with women who did not graduate from high school.[5] With respect to ethnic background, black and Hispanic women are more likely to rely on female sterilization, and white women are more likely to rely on an OCP.[1] Female sterilization is also the method most commonly relied on by women who are older than 34 years, have been married, or have a household income below 150% of the federal poverty line.[1]

Expressing and Discussing Contraceptive Efficacy

Contraceptive efficacy can be defined in many ways. Two terms used to express the number of unintended conceptions are the 'perfect-use' and 'typical-use' failure rates. The perfect-use failure rate is the number of conceptions that occur when the individual uses the method consistently and correctly (ie, perfectly) for 1 year. The individual may have used the contraceptive method previously, and the rate is determined for a year of continued use without a break in therapy. The typical-use failure rate is the number of conceptions that occur when the individual routinely uses a method in an inconsistent (eg, missing medication) or incorrect manner. This rate also assumes that the individual may have used the method before, and it is determined for a year of continued use.

A method's Pearl Index (PI) is defined as the number of unintended pregnancies/100 woman-years of method use. The PI is calculated by dividing the number of unintended pregnancies by the total number of woman-months or exposure cycles of observation and multiplying by 1,200 (for months) or by 1,300 (for cycles). The PI may underestimate the contraceptive efficacy because it is often based on a lengthy exposure interval, usually 1 year. Because contraceptive failure rates decline with use, long study intervals may not reflect contraceptive efficacy with short-term use.

Adolescent Patients

Sexual activity among adolescents in the United States is similar to that in other developed countries like Great Britain, France, Sweden, and Canada, but these countries have much lower pregnancy rates.[6] Between 1998 and 2001, teenagers in the United States were nearly twice as likely to become pregnant as teenagers in Great Britain and Canada and were three to four times more likely to become pregnant than teenagers in Sweden and France.

The lower conception rate in other countries is the result of higher rates of contraceptive use and, possibly, use of more effective methods. Teenagers aged 15 to 19 years in Great Britain, France, and Canada used OCPs twice as often as teenagers in the United States.

A recent report, however, suggests that younger adolescents are delaying sexual activity.[7] The proportion of never-married females aged 15 to 17 years who had ever had sexual intercourse dropped significantly from 38% in 1995 to 30% in 2002. For males aged 15 to 17 years, the percentage dropped significantly from 43% in 1995 to 31% in 2002. US teenagers were more likely to choose condoms for birth control when they became sexually active. Teenagers were also more likely to have used a contraceptive method at their most recent intercourse, 83% in 2002 compared with 71% in 1995.

There are many reasons why adolescents do not practice contraception or use less effective methods, including unavailability of services or an unwillingness to see a health-care provider. In a survey of adolescents attending a Planned Parenthood family planning clinic, half of the sexually active girls aged 12 to 17 years said they would stop attending the clinic if parents had to be notified.[8] Most of the same girls (57%) said they would switch to a less effective method or use no contraceptive method at all. Other reasons for inconsistent use and early discontinuation of a contraceptive method include the short duration of adolescent relationships[9]; failure to believe one might become pregnant, or ambivalence toward pregnancy[10,11]; and the presence or perception of side effects from the contraceptive method.[12]

References

1. Trussell J, Leveque JA, Koenig JD, et al: The economic value of contraception: a comparison of 15 methods. *Am J Public Health* 1995;85:494-503.

2. The Alan Guttmacher Institute: Facts in Brief: Contraceptive Use. Available at: http://www.guttmacher.org/pubs/fb_contr_use.html. Accessed February 26, 2007.

3. Chang J, Elam-Evans LD, Berg CJ, et al: Pregnancy-related mortality surveillance—United States, 1991-1999. *MMWR Surveill Summ* 2003;52:1-8.

4. Chiou CF, Trussell J, Reyes E, et al: Economic analysis of contraceptives for women. *Contraception* 2003;68:3-10.

5. Mosher WD, Martinez GM, Chandra A, et al: Use of contraception and use of family planning services in the United States: 1982-2002. Available at http://www.cdc.gov. Accessed February 26, 2007.

6. Darroch JE, Frost J, Singh S, et al: Teenage sexual and reproductive behavior in developed countries: can more progress be made? Available at: http://www.guttmacher.org/pubs/eurosynth_rpt.pdf. Accessed February 26, 2007.

7. National Center for Health Statistics: Teens delaying sexual activity: using contraception more effectively [press release]. Available at: http://www.cdc.gov/nchs/pressroom/04news/teens.htm. Accessed February 26, 2007.

8. Reddy DM, Fleming R, Swain C, et al: Effect of mandatory parental notification on adolescent girls' use of sexual health care services. *JAMA* 2002;288:710-714.

9. Manlove J, Ryan S, Franzetta K: Patterns of contraceptive use within teenagers' first sexual relationships. *Perspect Sex Reprod Health* 2003;35:246-255.

10. Crosby RA, Diclemente RJ, Wingood GM, et al: Adolescents' ambivalence about becoming pregnant predicts infrequent contraceptive use: a prospective analysis of nonpregnant African American females. *Am J Obstet Gynecol* 2002;186:251-252.

11. Jaccard J, Dodge T, Dittus P: Do adolescents want to avoid pregnancy? Attitudes toward pregnancy as predictors of pregnancy. *J Adolesc Health* 2003;33:79-83.

12. Rosenberg MJ, Waugh MS, Meehan TE: Use and misuse of oral contraceptives: risk indicators for poor pill taking and discontinuation. *Contraception* 1995;51:283-288.

Chapter 2

Steroid Contraception: Estrogen/Progestin Combination Oral Contraceptive Pills

Combination oral contraceptive pills (OCPs) are contraceptive medications that contain estrogen and progestin. They are the most prevalent form of reversible contraception used by US women aged 15 to 44 years. Approximately 10,410,000 US women use OCPs, or 26.9% of the total number of women using a contraceptive method.[1]

Estrogen Compounds

Two estrogen formulations have been consistently used in combination OCPs. The predominant estrogen in low-dose combination OCPs is ethinyl estradiol (EE). Mestranol (ethinyl estradiol 3-methyl ether), an estrogen found in older, high-dose combination OCPs, is metabolized to EE. EE is thought to be approximately 1.7 times stronger than mestranol.[2] A commonly accepted equivalence is that 50 µg of mestranol is similar to 30 µg of EE.[3]

The amount of estrogen used in OCPs has been steadily decreasing since the early formulations of the pill. The first OCP approved by the US Food and Drug Administration (FDA) was Enovid-10, which contained 150 µg of mestranol and 9.85 mg of norethynodrel. OCPs now have between 20 and 50 µg of EE for their estrogen component, which, compared with estrogen administration in menopause, is a pharmacologic range similar to the physiologic range of the reproductive years. An accepted conversion between EE and conjugated equine estrogen (CEE) is that 5 μg of EE is equivalent to 0.625 mg of CEE. Using a 20, 35, or 50 μg EE OCP would therefore be similar to taking 2.5, 4.375, or 6.5 mg of CEE/day. This amount of daily estrogen underscores the potential risk of thromboembolic events in women who are at increased risk or who use high-dose OCPs.

2

Progestin Compounds

While the estrogen component of combination OCPs is usually EE, the progestin formulation varies. Progestins are classified by their chemical structure (eg, 19-nortestosterone, 17-α spironolactone) or the time of their introduction to the market (ie, first, second, or third generation). These designations help to generalize the possible responses to a given OCP, but lowering the EE dose to decrease estrogen-related side effects can minimize progestin effects.

In the 19-nortestosterone group, the progestins are further divided into the estranes and the gonanes. The estranes are norethindrone (NET), norethindrone acetate (NETA), ethynodiol diacetate (ETD), lynestrenol, and norethynodrel. Estranes generally have a shorter half-life than the gonanes. NETA, ETD, lynestrenol, and norethynodrel are rapidly converted to NET, a portion of which undergoes further aromatization in hepatocytes to EE.[4] Previous work suggested that 1 mg of NETA was metabolized to 6 μg of EE, which could theoretically administer a substantial amount of EE (30 μg) from a standard 5 mg dose of NETA. A recent study by Lobo and colleagues[4a] has clarified this controversy and reduced the conversion of 1 mg of NETA to 2 μg of EE. Because of this hepatic aromatization, OCPs that use NET and NETA may be more estrogenic than their stated doses of EE.

The gonanes are norgestrel (NRG), levonorgestrel (LNG), desogestrel (DSG), norgestimate (NGM), and gestodene. Gestodene is not approved for use in the United

States. NRG is a racemic mixture of d-norgestrel and l-norgestrel (also known as levonorgestrel). The d- and l- notations refer to the ability of the steroid to rotate a plane of polarized light to the right (dextrorotatory) or the left (levorotatory), respectively. LNG is thus the active isomer of NRG. The gonanes have a longer half-life and greater progestational activity per unit weight than the estranes. This increased progestational activity allows for the use of a smaller amount of a gonane in an OCP formulation compared with an estrane progestin.

Drospirenone (DRSP) is the only available derivative of spironolactone. It has a longer half-life than other progestins of approximately 30 hours. DSRP retains some of spironolactone's inherent antimineralocorticoid and antiandrogenic activity. These properties are potentially helpful in decreasing androgenic side effects, but the FDA has recently reiterated that there is no substantial evidence that DRSP is more effective than other progestins and that the antimineralocorticoid activity may increase a patient's potassium level.[5] DRSP should not be used in patients with conditions that predispose them to hyperkalemia (ie, renal insufficiency, hepatic dysfunction, adrenal insufficiency). Certain drugs, when combined with DRSP, can increase the circulating serum potassium level. These medications include angiotensin-converting enzyme (ACE) inhibitors (Capoten®, Vasotec®, Zestril®), angiotensin II receptor antagonists (Avapro®, Cozaar®, Diovan®), potassium-sparing diuretics (spironolactone [Aldactone®]), heparin, aldosterone antagonists, and the long-term use of the nonsteroidal anti-inflammatory drugs ibuprofen (Advil®, Motrin®) and naproxen (Aleve®, Naprosyn®). If DRSP is to be used in patients taking these medications, the serum potassium level should be checked during the first OCP cycle.[6] The progestin DRSP is used in two OCPs, Yasmin® and YAZ®, containing 30 and 20 μg of EE, respectively. Both oral contraceptives are combined with 3 mg of the progestin DRSP.

Different progestins have different abilities to bind sex hormone-binding globulin (SHBG), but these differences are not clinically significant with regard to clinical parameters such as acne or hirsutism.[7,8] Attempts to determine whether one progestin is more or less androgenic than another in women based on animal studies (eg, growth of the rat ventral prostate) have not been successful. Because progestins have different effects at different end organs, a progestin's potency will vary depending on the end organ studied (eg, uterus, mammary gland). Any attempt to rank progestins with respect to potency or androgenicity is an exercise in futility. Differences among progestins in OCPs have been minimized as the estrogen doses have been lowered to be within the narrow range of 20 to 35 μg EE. In general, the amount of progestin in a pill formulation is set to oppose the estrogen's effect at the endometrium and prevent the luteinizing hormone (LH) surge. If the estrogen level is increased, a corresponding increase in progestin is necessary to maintain progestin dominance.

Contraceptive Mechanism and Efficacy

Estrogen and progestin inhibit at the level of the hypothalamus and at the pituitary gland,[9] blocking gonadotropin-releasing hormone (GnRH) and gonadotropin release (LH and follicle-stimulating hormone [FSH]), respectively. Despite GnRH infusion, women on OCPs demonstrate suppressed gonadotropin release. The progestin component primarily suppresses LH secretion, blocking ovulation, and the estrogen component suppresses FSH secretion, inhibiting folliculogenesis.[10] The progestin effect exceeds estrogen's effect at the level of the endometrium and cervix, leading to endometrial atrophy and thickened, hostile cervical mucus.[11] The estrogen component stabilizes the endometrium and decreases the incidence of atrophic breakthrough bleeding. Estrogen also increases the concentration of intracellular progestational receptors, which leads to a decrease in the overall OCP progestin dose.

The contraceptive failure rate for combination OCPs is approximately 0.3% in perfect use and 8% in typical use (see Appendix A). Several variables can lead to decreased contraceptive efficacy, including side effects, general noncompliance or poor adherence to the treatment regimen, increased body weight, and drug interactions that lead to increased metabolism of the steroid components.

The occurrence of side effects is often linked to early OCP discontinuation and subsequent contraceptive failure and unintended pregnancy. The occurrence of multiple side effects exponentially increases the likelihood of stopping OCP use. When one, two, or three side effects are present, the chance of OCP discontinuation is increased by 50%, 220%, or 320%, respectively.[12]

General noncompliance or poor adherence to the prescribed OCP treatment regimen includes starting a package of OCPs too late, missing pills, or taking a pill at different times each day. The importance of starting OCPs promptly after the onset of menses was highlighted in a research study that examined the initiation of OCP use at defined stages of ovarian follicular development.[13] The different stages of ovarian follicular development were based on the average diameter of the dominant follicle by transvaginal ultrasound scanning. In this study of 45 women who began their OCPs when the dominant follicle was 10, 14, or 18 mm in diameter, 0% (0/16 women), 36% (5/14 women), or 93% (14/15 women) of cycles were later ovulatory by serum progesterone measurement, respectively. The women were between the ages of 18 to 35, and they were suppressing ovulation with an OCP containing 30 μg of EE and 150 μg of DSG. The authors concluded that suppression of subsequent folliculogenesis by OCPs is closely tied to the diameter of the lead ovarian follicle. In the women starting their first OCP when the dominant follicle was 10 mm, the average day of pill initiation was 7.6 days, with a range of 1 to 16 days. Within the first 7 days of the menstrual cycle, the percentage of women with 10-, 14-, and 18-mm follicles were 45.5% (20/44 follicles), 6.9% (2/29 follicles), and 6.7% (1/15 follicles), respectively. These data would support the necessity of starting OCPs immediately after the 7-day pill-free interval. Women who start their OCPs after the traditional 7-day pill-free interval have an increased risk for a subsequent ovulatory cycle.

In a large European survey of 6,676 OCP users, Holt et al[14] examined the hypothesis that greater body weight increases the risk of OCP failure. They assessed the relative risk (RR) of pregnancy for women weighing ≥155 pounds and found that the RR of contraceptive failure was 60% greater in women who weighed >155 pounds compared with women who weighed less (RR=1.6; 95% CI 1.1, 2.4). For women who weighed at least 155 pounds, the risk of unintended pregnancy was greater when using an OCP containing 20 to 30 μg EE (RR=4.5; 95% CI 1.4, 14.4) compared with an OCP containing ≤35 μg EE (RR=2.6; 95% CI 1.2, 5.9). These findings suggest that contraceptive efficacy is decreased in women who weigh ≥155 pounds and that a dose of 20 to 30 μg EE may be less effective than a dose of ≤35 μg EE in these women. The effect of body weight on contraceptive efficacy has become more important as the average body weight of US women has steadily increased since 1960. In the latest (1999-2002) National Health and Nutrition Examination Survey (NHANES), the average weight of women 20 years and older was 163 pounds, an increase of 10 pounds over the average weight in the 1994-1998 survey.[15]

Some medications, when used concomitantly with OCPs, can increase the metabolism of OCP steroids, leading to decreased contraceptive efficacy. These medications are listed in the section 'Drug Interactions With Combination OCPs' below.

Traditional Use of OCPs

Traditionally, combination OCPs are ingested for 3 weeks, followed by an intervening week of placebo tablets. Some placebo tablets are 'reminder' or 'inert' pills, while some contain 75 mg of ferrous fumarate (eg, Estrostep® Fe, Loestrin® 24 Fe, Loestrin® Fe 1.5/30, Loestrin® Fe 1/20, and their generic equivalents). The purpose of the week off is to allow a steroid withdrawal uterine bleeding that simulates a menstrual period similar to a nonconception spontaneous ovulatory cycle. The presence of a monthly menses is perceived as making the OCP regimen as 'natural' or as close to a woman's regular menstrual pattern as possible. An absence of bleeding suggests a contraceptive failure and conception during the recent cycle of medication.

OCP Formulations

Combination OCPs are often classified as either monophasic or multiphasic (see Appendix D). These terms refer to whether the estrogen and/or progestin level is constant (monophasic) or changes within the pack of OCPs (multiphasic). Monophasic pills were developed first, followed by multiphasic pills. The rationale for an alteration in the steroid dose was to minimize side effects. Below are representative examples of different pill formulations available in the United States.

Monophasic Pills

Femcon® Fe (Warner Chilcott)
http://www.femconfe.com
Toll-free telephone number: 1-800-521-8813
Ortho-Novum® 1/35
(Ortho-McNeil Pharmaceutical, Inc.)
http://orthowomenshealth.com
Toll-free telephone number : 1-877-323-2200

These two monophasic preparations use 35 μg of EE and different doses of NET. In Femcon® Fe, the NET is a constant 0.4 mg/pill (Figure 2-1). In the Ortho-Novum® 1/35 formulation, a higher dose of NET, 1 mg, is present in each pill (Figure 2-2). There are 21 steroid-containing pills, followed by seven iron tablets (Femcon® Fe) or seven inactive pills (Ortho-Novum® 1/35).

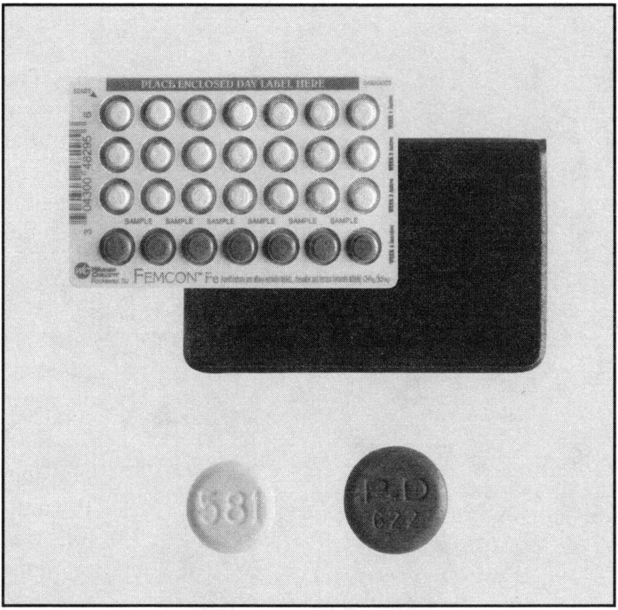

Figure 2-1: Femcon® Fe (monophasic pill).

The Ortho-Novum® 1/35 and Femcon® Fe pills are comparable because they both contain EE and NET. However, the Femcon® Fe formulation has the lowest effective dose of NET (0.4 mg) combined with 35 μg of EE, which provides exceptional cycle control with minimal breakthrough bleeding. With this minimal amount of progestin, Femcon® Fe is one of the most estrogenic of all the 35 μg EE OCPs available. It is an excellent choice for the woman with hirsutism and acne (as seen in women with polycystic ovarian syndrome, see 'Selecting an OCP' section below). The simplicity of its monophasic design makes it an excellent choice for patients initiating OCPs and allows it to be used in an off-label, extended fashion (see 'Alterations of the Combination OCP Method' below).

Lake Superior College Library

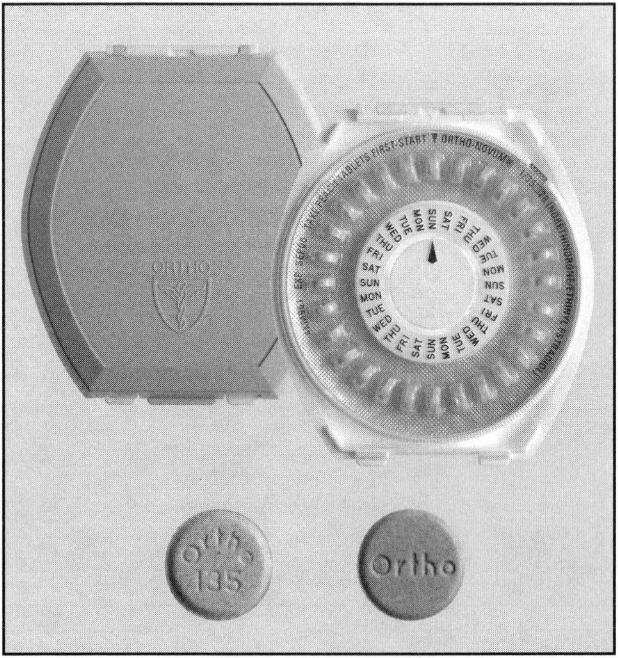

Figure 2-2: Ortho-Novum® 1/35 (monophasic pill).

In addition, Femcon® Fe is the only OCP available that can be chewed and swallowed as well as swallowed whole. Although the package insert instructs women to drink 8 ounces (240 mL) of water after taking Femcon® Fe, similar average circulating concentrations of EE and NET have been reported in women who chewed the pill and swallowed a similar pill (same doses of EE and NET) and did not drink water after pill ingestion.[16] The flexibility of ingesting an OCP with or without water may improve the chances of consuming a pill daily and decrease side effects. Femcon® Fe is a chewable spearmint-flavored OCP that is more convenient and offers an easy-to-use option over the traditional swallowed pill.

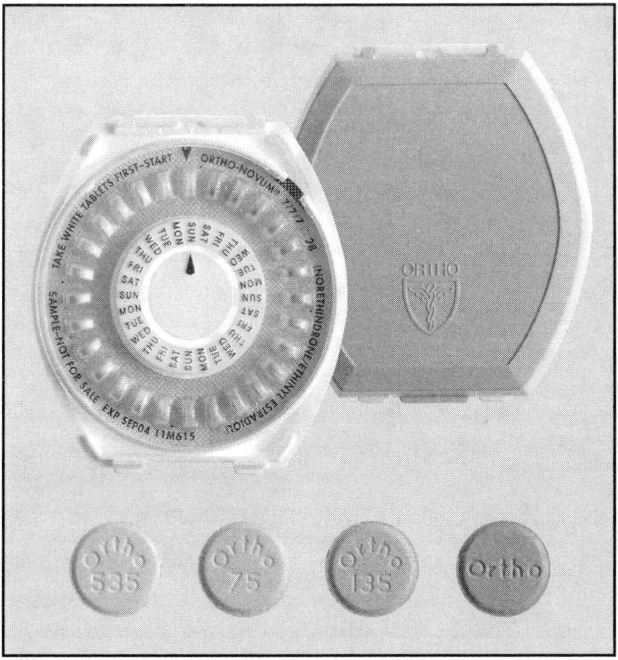

Figure 2-3: Ortho-Novum® 7/7/7 (multiphasic pill with graduated progestin dose).

Multiphasic Pills: Alteration in Progestin Dose

Ortho-Novum® 7/7/7
(Ortho-McNeil Pharmaceutical, Inc.)
http://orthowomenshealth.com
Toll-free telephone number : 1-877-323-2200

In one of the first multiphasic pills, Ortho-Novum® 7/7/7, the progestin dose of NET was lowered in the initial 14 pills to decrease the overall progestin dose administered during a cycle of medication. Instead of a constant dose of 1 mg of NET, the amount of NET is decreased to 0.5 mg/pill for the first 7 days, increased to 0.75 mg/pill for 7 days, and returned to a 1 mg/pill dose of NET for the last 7 days (Figure 2-3). This

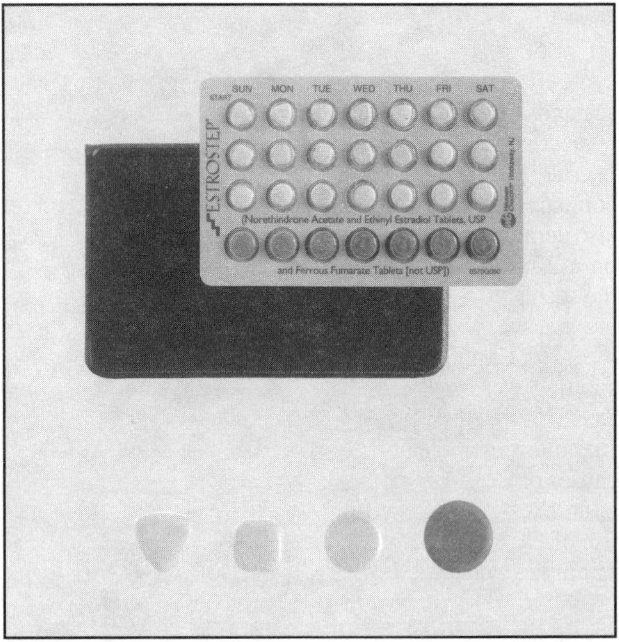

Figure 2-4: Estrostep® Fe (multiphasic pill with graduated estrogen dose).

overall lower dose of progestin decreases progestin-mediated side effects early in the cycle of pill administration.

Multiphasic OCPs: Alteration in Estrogen Dose

Estrostep® Fe(Warner Chilcott)
http://www.estrostep.com
Toll-free telephone number: 1-800-521-8813

To decrease estrogen-related side effects early in the cycle and reduce the incidence of breakthrough bleeding and spotting in the last 2 weeks of pill administration, Estrostep® Fe uses a graduated, increasing dose of estrogen: 5 days of 20 μg EE, 7 days of 30 μg EE, and 9 days of 35 μg EE (Figure 2-4). The progestin dose remains a constant 1 mg of NETA. In a study of 690 women using a 20, 30, or 50 μg EE or a graduated estrogen dose OCP for 4 cycles, the average percentage of women reporting nausea and/or vomiting was 1.35%, 2.2%, 5.1%, and 0.92%, respectively.[17] The graduated estrogen dose formulation markedly reduced the occurrence of nausea and vomiting compared with the monophasic preparations. This study also demonstrated that breakthrough bleeding and spotting on a 20 μg EE monophasic OCP occurred primarily in the second and third weeks of pill administration. When a graduated estrogen dose formulation was compared with the 20 μg EE monophasic OCP, breakthrough bleeding and spotting were reduced to levels lower than those associated with a 30 or 50 μg EE monophasic OCP. Bleeding irregularities and nausea are the two most frequently cited causes of OCP discontinuation.[18] Estrostep® Fe, therefore, is an excellent choice for women who are initiating the use of OCPs or who are already using OCPs and want to minimize side effects.

Contraindications to Combination OCPs

Almost all the contraindications to combination OCPs are secondary to the pharmacologic level of estrogen.[19] They include (1) a history of thrombophlebitis, thromboembolic disorders, cerebrovascular disease, or coronary occlusion; (2) severely impaired liver function; (3) known or suspected breast cancer; (4) unexplained vaginal bleeding; (5) known or suspected pregnancy; (6) tobacco smoking (in women older than 35 years); (7) severe hypercholesterolemia or hypertriglyceridemia; and (8) uncontrolled hypertension.

Side Effects

The occurrence of side effects is the most important factor associated with the discontinuation of oral contraceptives.[12] Common side effects cited as reasons for OCP discontinuation are weight gain, nausea, headache,

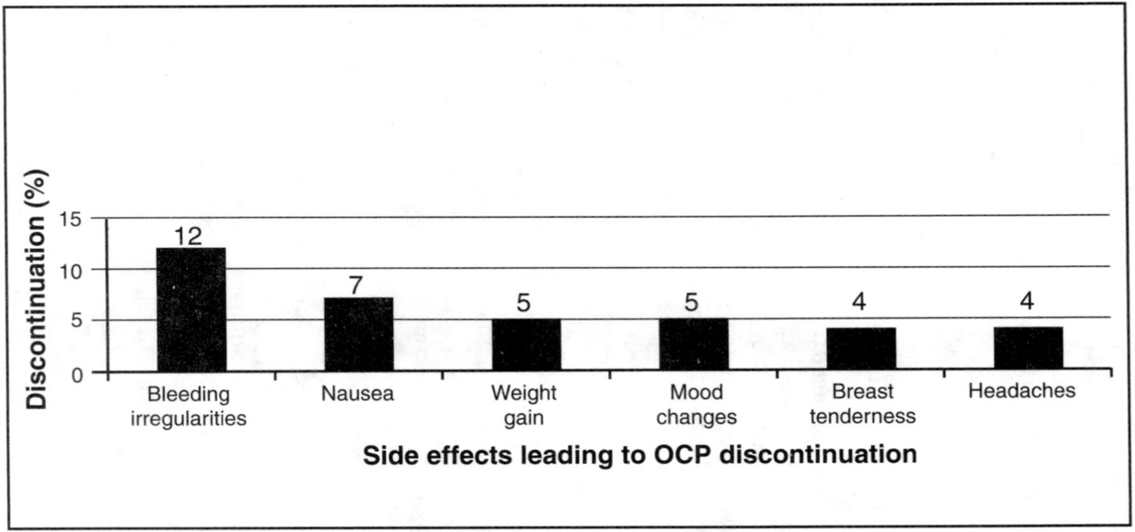

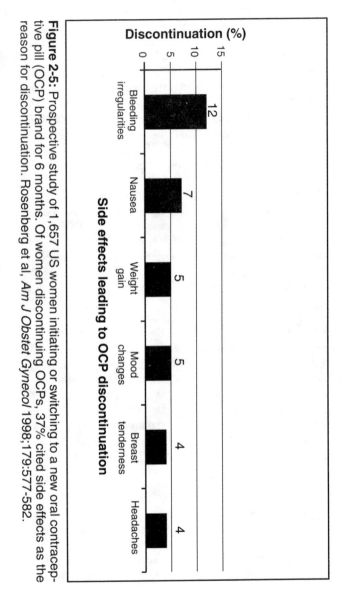

Figure 2-5: Prospective study of 1,657 US women initiating or switching to a new oral contraceptive pill (OCP) brand for 6 months. Of women discontinuing OCPs, 37% cited side effects as the reason for discontinuation. Rosenberg et al, *Am J Obstet Gynecol* 1998;179:577-582.

and menstrual abnormalities. In one national survey of US women, the single most commonly cited side effect leading to OCP discontinuation was weight gain during pill use (11%).[20] However, this survey encompassed OCP use between the years of 1973 and 1982, when higher-dose OCPs (>35 μg EE) were more prevalent. In a more recent prospective study of 128 women using a 35 μg EE triphasic OCP, there was no significant weight gain over 4 cycles of OCP use.[21] Most women (52%) remained within 2 pounds (0.9 kg) of their starting weight, and 72% had no weight gain or loss. The women were weighed daily. The mean weight rose one-half pound (0.2 kg) during the first 2 weeks of the cycle and then fell to baseline during the last few days of the cycle. The perception of weight gain during OCP use seems to be partly caused by inherent weight fluctuations during the cycle. Patients should be advised of these small weight changes and the lack of overall weight gain with a 35 μg EE OCP. However, the perception that OCPs cause weight gain has affected a generation of pill users, and their experience may influence younger pill users' choice of contraceptive methods.

In a prospective study of 1,657 US women initiating or switching to a new OCP brand for 6 months, questionnaires were collected from 1,062 (64.9%) and 887 (53.5%) of women at 2 and 6 months, respectively, for the analysis of discontinuation rates and the appearance of side effects on OCPs.[18] The study was conducted from March 1995 to May 1996 and used primarily 30 and 35 μg EE OCPs. Eleven percent of women discontinued OCP use after the first cycle, and 4% discontinued in the second cycle. Another 13% of women discontinued OCP use during the next 4 cycles. Of the 293 women who discontinued OCP use, the largest group, 37%, cited side effects as responsible for their discontinuation (Figure 2-5). The side effects cited were bleeding irregularities (12%), nausea (7%), weight gain (5%), mood changes (5%), breast tenderness (4%), and headaches (4%).

Patients who smoke have a higher frequency of vaginal spotting and bleeding than nonsmokers, possibly because estrogen is catabolized by nicotine, leading to general hypoestrogenism and less estrogenic support of the endometrium. In a study by Rosenberg et al,[22] cigarette smokers were 47% more likely to have vaginal spotting or bleeding than nonsmokers during 6 cycles of OCP use. By the sixth cycle, women who smoked (>16 cigarettes/day) were almost 3 (2.92) times more likely to have vaginal spotting or bleeding than nonsmokers. Women who smoke cigarettes should be alerted to the increased frequency of this side effect, which may lead to early discontinuation and dissatisfaction with combination OCPs.

Alterations of the Combination OCP Method

Combination OCP Dosing Regimens

Mircette® (Barr Laboratories, Inc.)
http://www.mircette.com
Kariva® (Barr Laboratories, Inc.)
http://www.barrlabs.com
Toll-free telephone number: 1-800-222-4043

There have been attempts to alter the number of pill-free interval days. One 20 μg EE OCP, Mircette®, is formulated for 21 days of active pills, followed by 2 days of placebo and 5 days of 10 μg EE. The rationale for this formulation is to limit the number of days of hypoestrogenism after 21 days of active pills. It was anticipated that the 5 days of unopposed estrogen would prevent FSH from rising and prevent early folliculogenesis during the usual 7-day placebo period. A prospective, randomized, double-blind study of the Mircette® OCP vs the same active pill regimen with a 7-day placebo pill interval revealed a greater degree of ovarian suppression with the 2 days of placebo and 5 days of 10 μg EE compared with the 7-day placebo formulation.[23] It was also anticipated that users would have fewer estrogen-withdrawal headaches during the shorter

2-day placebo period. In an 18-month, open-label, multicenter Mircette® study of 1,143 women (1,080.8 woman-years of use), the Pearl Index for total pregnancies during treatment was 1.02/100 woman-years. In the study, 43.9% of women reported drug-related side effects, of which the most common was headache.[24]

Loestrin® 24 Fe (Warner Chilcott)
http://www.warnerchilcott.com
http://www.shortperiod.com
Toll-free telephone number: 1-800-521-8813

To decrease the number of days of menstrual bleeding and improve contraceptive efficacy, three additional 20 μg EE-containing active OCPs were added to the existing Loestrin® 1/20 formulation, creating a 28-day pill pack with 24 active and 4 iron pills (Figure 2-6). This strategy of shortening the placebo interval is especially important for women entering the perimenopause period of their lives. In perimenopause, there is increased FSH secretion during the placebo interval that shortens the follicular phase of the menstrual cycle. By shortening the placebo interval from 7 days to 4 days, there is less chance for an oocyte (egg) to develop and lead to an unintended ovulation. In a randomized comparison between Loestrin® 24 Fe and Loestrin® 21 1/20, the 21-day active pill formulation, a total of 938 women were randomized (751 and 187, respectively) for a 6-month study.[25] This study was performed in women 18 to 45 years; 83% were ≤35 years and 17% were >35 years. Women with a history of cigarette smoking were allowed to enroll unless they were older than 35 years and smoked >15 cigarettes/day. Other study inclusion criteria included a body mass index (BMI) of ≤35 kg/m^2 and a willingness to use the study medication as the only form of contraception. The study sought to examine primarily young women, and the inclusion criteria allowed for a wide range of body weights. With respect to contraceptive efficacy, the Pearl Index was 1.82 (95% CI 0.59-4.25) in the Loestrin® 24 Fe for all subjects and 1.79 (95% CI 0.49-4.57) for subjects

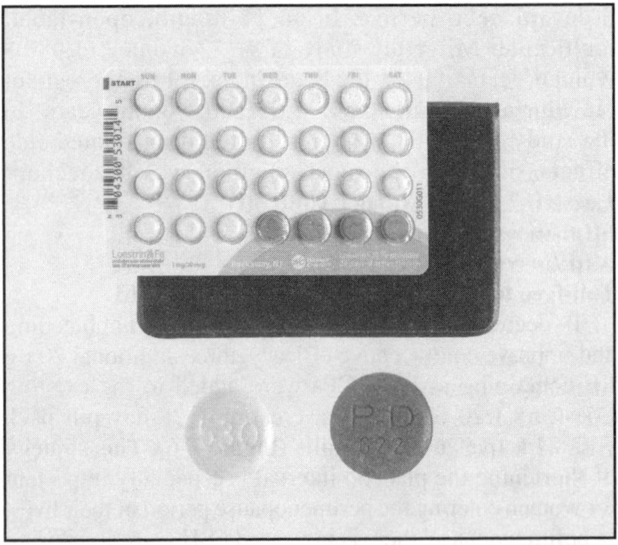

Figure 2-6: Loestrin® 24 Fe (24 days of active pills and 4 days of iron pills).

≤35 years. In comparison, the Pearl Index was 2.98 for all subjects using the Loestrin® Fe 1/20. The cumulative risk of pregnancy in the first 6 months of Loestrin® 24 Fe was 0.9% (determined by Kaplan-Meier life-table analysis). Although the decrease in the pregnancy rate was not statistically significant, this study was not powered to test for a difference in treatment efficacy. In contrast to other OCP contraceptive efficacy studies, these studies often determine the Pearl Index in a selected group of women in a noncomparative fashion. In the current study, the lower Pearl Index determined for Loestrin® 24 Fe compared with Loestrin® Fe 1/20 provides a clinically useful evaluation of the contraceptive efficacy since it estimates the pregnancy rate in the same population randomized to the two different products in a head-to-head comparison. In terms of menstrual withdrawal bleeding, the period length was noted to decrease significantly starting as early as cycle 2 and continuing through cycle 6. By the sixth cycle of Loestrin® 24 Fe use, the average period length was 2.66 days compared with 3.88 days for Loestrin® Fe 1/20. This difference (>1 day of less bleeding) was statistically significant, 2.66 vs 3.88 days, *P* <0.001. With Loestrin® 24 Fe, there was also less intracycle (breakthrough) bleeding compared with Loestrin® Fe 1/20 that became statistically significantly less by the sixth cycle of Loestrin® 24 Fe use (0.95 vs 1.63 days, respectively, *P*=0.005).

YAZ® (Berlex, Inc.)
http://www.yaz-us.com
Toll-free telephone number:
1-888-BERLEX-4, (1-888-237-5394)

Shortly after the introduction of Loestrin® 24 Fe, YAZ® was introduced in the United States in April 2006. YAZ® also has 24 days of a combination estrogen/progestin medication, 20 µg of EE and 3 mg of DRSP, respectively, followed by 4 days of inert placebo tablets. An open-label, noncomparative, efficacy and safety study of YAZ® determined that the Pearl Index for OCP was 1.29 (upper limit of the 95% CI 2.3) and cumulative 1-year pregnancy rate (determined by Kaplan-Meier life-table analysis) was 1.26% (95% CI 0.52-2.01).[26]

Studies have been performed to determine whether YAZ® would be effective against premenstrual dysphoric disorder (PMDD). In an initial double-blind study of 449 women, 231 and 218 were randomized to YAZ® and placebo, respectively.[26] The subjects were studied for three treatment cycles. Of the subjects randomized, 161 (69.4%) and 167 (76.6%) completed the study in the YAZ® and placebo group, respectively. YAZ® improved symptoms of PMDD, with the greatest improvement in physical symptoms (ie, breast tenderness, swelling, bloating, headache, muscle pain), adjusted mean difference of -1.4 (95% CI -2.11 to -0.77), *P* <0.001. In a more rigorous but smaller study, Pearlstein and colleagues[27] conducted a randomized, double-blind, placebo-controlled, crossover design study consisting of three cycles of YAZ® or placebo followed by a washout cycle and three cycles of the remaining treatment. Of the 64 subjects randomized, only 23 completed the study (36%)—14 YAZ®/placebo and 9 placebo/YAZ®. YAZ® improved symptoms of PMDD, with the greatest improvement in physical symptoms (ie, breast tenderness, swelling, bloating, headache, muscle pain), adjusted mean difference of -2.5, P=0.003. These studies led to YAZ® receiving FDA approval for the treatment of the emotional and physical symptoms of PMDD in October 2006.

In sharp contrast, however, in a double-blind, placebo-controlled study using Yasmin® (30 μg EE and 3 mg DRSP, 21 days of active and 7 days of placebo pills) in 82 women with PMDD, Yasmin® failed to demonstrate significant improvement over placebo therapy for treatment of PMDD symptoms.[28] The explanation for the apparent difference in results between Yasmin® and YAZ® may be the result of greater progestin dominance in YAZ® (the same 3 mg of DRSP opposing only 20 μg rather than 30 μg of EE in YAZ® and Yasmin®, respectively) and/or because of a shortening of the pill-free interval from 7 to 4 days of placebo pills. A shorter pill-free interval leads to less ovarian folliculogenesis and less endogenous hormone expression.[29] Stabilization of both endogenous and exogenous hormone levels from OCPs may lead to less PMDD symptom expression.[30] Since the two YAZ® PMDD studies were performed only against placebo tablets and not another OCP, similar results might be expected from other OCPs with a shortened pill-free interval. Similarly, since all OCPs alter intracycle and withdrawal menstrual bleeding, these symptoms can unblind both enrolled subjects and study investigators, leading to biased study results.

In comparison with Yasmin®, YAZ® is more progestin dominant. Both have 3 mg of DRSP, but, in YAZ®, the progestin dose is only opposing 20 μg of EE rather than 30 μg of EE in Yasmin®. Because of the progestin dominance, one may see more progestin side effects (ie, bloating, breast discomfort, weight gain, fatigue) with YAZ® than with Yasmin®. Similar to Yasmin®, YAZ® uses 3 mg of DRSP, which is comparable with 25 mg of spironolactone. The package insert for YAZ® recommends checking a patient's serum potassium level if the OCP is combined with ACE inhibitors (Capoten®, Vasotec®, Zestril®), angiotensin II receptor antagonists (Avapro®, Cozaar®, Diovan®), potassium-sparing diuretics (spironolactone), heparin, aldosterone antagonists, and long-term use of nonsteroidal anti-inflammatory drugs, ibuprofen (Advil®, Motrin®), and naproxen (Aleve®, Naprosyn®). DRSP-containing OCPs should not be used by patients with conditions that predispose them to hyperkalemia (ie, renal insufficiency, hepatic dysfunction, adrenal insufficiency).

Other Combination OCP Dosing Regimens Not Currently Available in the United States

Two other 20 μg EE OCP formulations, a 23-day[31] and a 24-day[32] active pill regimen have been reported, but they are not available for clinical use in the United States. In the 23-day formulation, which contains 75 μg of gestodene, estradiol levels during the last 6 days of the cycle and the first 6 days of the next cycle were significantly less ($P < 0.05$) than those associated with a similar 21-day formulation, suggesting greater suppression of ovarian activity.

Extended or Continuous Dosing of Combined OCPs

Recent research studies have questioned the usefulness of a monthly withdrawal menses and have let patients select the number of weeks to ingest their combination OCPs.[33,34] The purposes of adding additional weeks of medication were to delay hormone withdrawal symptoms and to allow patients to have fewer menstrual periods per year. Extended-dose OCP regimens usually vary between 3 and 12 weeks. Patients have combined two, three, or four traditional OCP packs to ingest medication for 6, 9, or 12 weeks, respectively. One combination OCP brand, Seasonale®, packages an active pill with 30 μg EE OCP and 0.15 mg LNG in a 13-week dispenser pack, containing 12 weeks of active medication followed by 7 days of inert placebo pills.

Although the concept of having only four withdrawal menses per year is attractive to some patients, this discrete bleeding pattern is not initially achieved. Patients who initiate Seasonale® without using OCPs in the preceding 28 days will experience more breakthrough vaginal bleeding and spotting than if they had used the same medication for 3 weeks followed by an intervening placebo week for 4 treatment cycles.[35] In a comparative trial, 65% of women using Seasonale® had 7 or more days of bleeding in their first 12 weeks of medication compared with 38% of women using the same formulation for 3 weeks followed by a 1-week placebo period for 4 treatment cycles (Table 2-1). During 1 year of treatment, the bleeding profile on the fourth cycle of Seasonale® was similar to that of women using the same formulation in a traditional regimen during cycles 10 through 13 (Table 2-1). The initial increased vaginal bleeding is highlighted in the product's full prescribing information.

The use of a traditional OCP regimen (21 days of active pills followed by 7 pill-free interval days) allows for gradual atrophy of the endometrium and timed withdrawal menstrual bleeding. A patient who chooses to institute an extended-dose OCP regimen will have less breakthrough bleeding if she has used OCPs in a traditional regimen before extending the number of active pills to 6, 9, or 12 weeks. This period of timed withdrawal bleeding will allow the endometrium to atrophy, and there will be less breakthrough bleeding when she switches to an extended-dose regimen.

Some clinicians instruct their patients to ingest their OCPs daily or 'continuously' until they have vaginal bleeding. This type of bleeding is attributed to extreme atrophy of the endometrium, with intermittent breakdown of the thin endometrial lining, and is thought to be secondary to the prolonged exposure of the endometrium to the progestin component of the OCP. The bleeding is characteristically a

Table 2-1: Intermenstrual Bleeding in Women Using Seasonale® vs 28-Day-Cycle Pill*

Days of Intermenstrual Bleeding and/or Spotting	Percentage of Subjects**	
Seasonale®	***Cycle 1***	***Cycle 4***
7 or more days	65%	42%
20 or more days	35%	15%
28-day-cycle pill	***Cycles 1-4***	***Cycles 10-13***
7 or more days	38%	39%
20 or more days	6%	4%

* Dosage of 28-day-cycle pill was equivalent to that of Seasonale®.

** Based on bleeding and/or spotting on days 1 through 84 of a 91-day cycle in Seasonale® subjects and days 1 through 21 of a 28-day cycle over 4 cycles in subjects using a 28-day dosing regimen. Seasonale® prescribing information. Barr Laboratories, Inc., Pomona, NY, 2003.

dark brownish discharge of old menstrual blood. It occurs variably, sometimes starting in as early as 6 to 9 weeks of OCP use. Patients are instructed to stop taking OCPs for 1 week while they are having atrophic vaginal bleeding and then restart their medication on a daily basis until vaginal bleeding occurs again.

Progestin-related side effects of continuous OCP use include breast fullness or hardness, abdominal bloating, general fatigue, and decreased libido. These symptoms subside when the OCPs are discontinued for 3 to 7 days. Because vaginal bleeding can be caused by patient noncompliance (eg, forgetting to take the pill, running out of medication prematurely), it is helpful to choose a set duration of pill use (eg, 6, 9, or 12 weeks) usually based on the number of OCP packs taken continuously. Persistent vaginal bleeding at times other than the placebo week can be investigated with a vaginal ultrasound examination with or without saline infusion enhancement or office hysteroscopy. Sometimes endometrial polyps are responsible for the vaginal bleeding. If the endometrium is thin, 3 to 5 mm in thickness, and uniform without evidence of polyps, then progestin-mediated atrophy is the likely etiology. Endometrial atrophy will respond to the administration of supplemental estrogen given with the OCPs for 7 to 14 days. Upon stopping the additional estrogen and OCPs, a withdrawal menses ensues. After 7 days, OCP use can be restarted. The supplemental estrogen can be given orally (0.625 to 1.25 mg of CEE), or an equivalent amount can be given by either a transdermal or a vaginal route of administration. If a vaginal route is chosen, approximately 25% to 50% less estrogen can be given to achieve the desired effect.[36]

After the initial increased breakthrough bleeding rates, irregular bleeding will return to baseline at approximately 10 months of successful extended OCP use, and there will be decreased menstrual flow at the time of anticipated menses (Table 2-1). In women using the Seasonale® OCP, endometrial biopsies after 1 year of therapy revealed inactive or atrophic endometrium, demonstrating the progestin effect at the lining of the uterus.[37]

In an effort to decrease unscheduled (breakthrough) vaginal bleeding associated with the Seasonale® OCP, a modification was made replacing the seven inert placebos with seven 10 μg EE pills. This new OCP, Seasonique™, retains the same 13-week dispenser pack now containing 12 weeks of active medication (30 μg of EE and 0.15 mg of LNG) followed by seven 10 μg EE pills. In an open-label efficacy study,[38] 708 women ages 18 to 35 were treated in 2,177 extended-regimen 91-day cycles. The Pearl Index in all treated subjects with at least one 91-day cycle was 1.27. The cumulative failure rate at the end of 1 year of treatment, estimated by Kaplan-Meier life-table analysis in all treated subjects, was 0.61%. There were no pregnancies in women weighing >90 kg. In the same study, scheduled (withdrawal) and unscheduled (breakthrough) bleeding and/or spotting decreased during the 12-month study period (Table 2-2). The addition of 10 μg of unopposed EE for 7 days may stimulate the atrophic endometrium and lead to less unscheduled breakthrough bleeding. In subjects using Seasonique™ compared with Seasonale®,[39] there appears to be less unscheduled breakthrough bleeding in subjects using Seasonique™ (Table 2-2). Although the study populations for the two studies were not identical, they were similar in design and both used an electronic diary to record the subject's bleeding patterns. Because of the limited amount of available information on the cycle-specific Seasonale® bleeding pattern, only the median number of unscheduled bleeding/spotting days is available to compare with Seasonique™ (Table 2-2).

Quick-Start Initiation of OCPs

To prevent delay and possible confusion about when to start OCP use, some investigators have used a same-day 'quick start' approach to initiating OCPs.[40,41] A quick start differs from starting on the first day of menses or on the Sunday after the next menses (termed a Sunday start) by starting OCPs on the day that the patient is seen in the office, regardless of the day of her menstrual cycle. A negative urine pregnancy test is obtained during the patient's office visit, and the patient is given an OCP to ingest in the office. If there is a recent history of unprotected exposure to sperm, emergency contraceptive medication can be given. The patient is given a sample pack of OCPs to use, to avoid requiring her to stop at a pharmacy. A benefit of the quick-start method is that it avoids having the patient use a less-effective or less-acceptable temporary contraceptive method before her next menses.

In a prospective observational cohort study of 250 women, in which a quick-start approach was compared

Table 2-2: Scheduled (Withdrawal) and Unscheduled (Breakthrough) Bleeding/Spotting Days in Women Using Seasonale® and Seasonique™

Cycle	Scheduled Bleeding/Spotting: Seasonique™[38] Mean (SD) per Cycle	Median
1	3.4 (2.1)	3
2	3.1 (2.1)	3
3	2.8 (2)	3
4	2.8 (2)	3

with initiating OCPs at any other time before the next menses (a delayed start after the patient's initial visit), quick-start patients were significantly more likely to use their second pack of OCPs 6 weeks after their initial visit (adjusted odds ratio [OR]=2.8; 95% CI 1.1, 7.3).[41] In a retrospective cohort chart review of 193 women ≤22 years, those who used the quick-start method (n=77) were more likely to still be using OCPs 3 months after initiation than those who used a Sunday start (72% vs 56%, *P*=0.059).[40] The quick-start users were more likely to comply at 3 months if they were white (80% vs 65%, *P*=0.007), had dysmenorrhea (86% vs 62%, *P*=0.006), were nulligravid (77% vs 58%, *P*=0.008), or were nulliparous (73% vs 59%, *P*=0.038).

Fetal exposure to OCPs is not thought to be harmful.[42] The vaginal bleeding profile of quick-start users is no different from that of users who initiate their OCPs after their initial visit and before their next menses.

2

Cycle	Unscheduled Bleeding/Spotting		
	Seasonique™[38]		Seasonale®[39]
	Mean (SD) per Cycle	*Median*	*Median*
1	14.3 (13.6)	11	12
2	9.5 (10.5)	5	6
3	7.2 (9)	5	6
4	7.6 (9.4)	4	4

General Considerations When Using Combination OCPs

Effect on the Cardiovascular System

There are two types of thrombosis: venous thromboembolism (VTE) and arterial thrombosis. VTE is characterized by low flow, high fibrinogen, and a low platelet count and appears clinically as either deep vein thrombosis (DVT) or pulmonary embolism. Arterial thrombosis is characterized by high flow, low fibrinogen, and a high platelet count. It appears clinically as either myocardial infarction (MI) or stroke.

Because of their pharmacologic levels of estrogen, OCPs increase the production of clotting factors, which in turn increases the risk of VTE.[43] When compared with pregnancy, however, the use of OCPs is 2 to 6 times less likely to lead to a nonfatal VTE event.[44,45] In general, low-dose combination OCPs (≤35 μg EE) do not appreciably affect the cardiovascular system in healthy women <35 years who

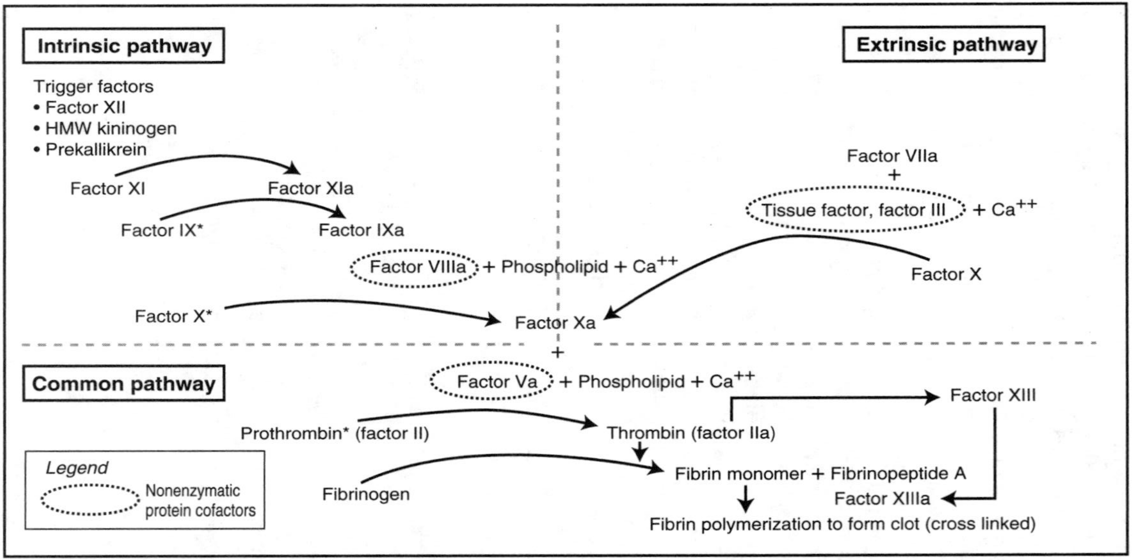

Figure 2-7: Blood coagulation cascade. HMW=high molecular weight. *=activated on phospholipid surfaces, a=activated.

do not smoke cigarettes.[19] Women who have risk factors for hypercoagulability or who are ≥35 years and smoke cigarettes are at increased risk and should not use OCPs.[46] Once OCPs are discontinued, past users do not have an increased incidence of cardiovascular disease.[47]

Blood Coagulation Cascade

The blood coagulation cascade exists to generate thrombin (activated factor II, factor IIa), which converts the soluble plasma protein fibrinogen to insoluble fibrin monomer and the cleavage products fibrinopeptide A and B. The fibrin monomer polymerizes when exposed to activated factor XIII (XIIIa) to form fibrin clots. Figure 2-7 shows the intrinsic, extrinsic, and common pathways of coagulation.

As a safeguard against excessive thrombosis, the entire cascade is balanced by natural anticoagulants in the body. These anticoagulants are antithrombin III, which inhibits the intrinsic pathway; protein C and protein S, which inhibit the formation of factors V and VIII; and tissue plasminogen activator (t-PA), which converts plasminogen to plasmin, which then degrades fibrin and lyses clots.

Hemostasis is affected by a number of coagulation parameters, including platelet count, prothrombin time, activated partial thromboplastin time, antithrombin III activity, fibrinogen, and fibrinopeptide A levels. Hemostasis can also be affected by vasodilators and vasoconstrictors that mediate vascular tone. Prostacyclin is a potent vasodilator and an inhibitor of platelet aggregation. It is opposed by a potent vasoconstrictor, thromboxane A_2 (TXA_2), which increases platelet aggregation and adhesiveness.

Effect of OCPs and Cigarette Smoking on the Coagulation System

In a 9-month prospective study of three low-dose (≤35 μg EE) OCPs, there was an increase in clotting factors and platelet activity, denoting an increased risk for VTE.[43] Estrogen increases hepatic production of serum globulins (clotting factors) involved in coagulation. Specifically, procoagulant activity is increased as the result of a 10%

Table 2-3: Coagulation Parameters in Tobacco Smokers and Nonsmokers Using Combination Oral Contraceptive Pills

	35 μg EE	
	NS	**S**
Fibrinogen	↑	↑
Fibrinopeptide A	↑	↑
Prothrombin time		↑
Antithrombin III activity	↑	

EE=ethinyl estradiol, NS=nonsmokers, S=smokers
Fruzzetti et al: *Contraception* 1994;49:579-592.

to 20% increase in fibrinogen, increased factor VII and X levels, and a twofold increase in fibrinopeptide A levels.[48,49] The occurrence of VTE appears to be estrogen dependent, and OCPs with higher doses of estrogen (50 μg EE) have an increased risk for VTE compared with lower-dose OCPs.[47] This risk diminishes and returns to normal about 3 months after OCPs are discontinued.[47] The baseline risk for VTE in healthy women is reported to be 4 cases/100,000 women. The use of a low-dose (≤35 μg EE) OCP is thought to increase the risk of VTE to 10 to 15 cases/100,000 women, but the risk from pregnancy is higher (60 cases/100,000 women).[45] Another comparative study estimated the incidence of VTE/100,000 woman-years to be approximately 10 for women who did not use OCPs, 30 for low-dose OCP users, and 60 for pregnant women.[44]

When OCP use is accompanied by cigarette smoking, there is an increased risk for thrombosis because of a

30 μg EE		20 μg EE	
NS	S	NS	S
	↑		
↑	↑		
			↑

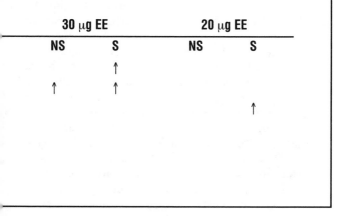

nicotine-mediated decrease in circulating prostacyclin and an increase in thromboxane levels, leading to increased platelet aggregation.[50] Fruzzetti et al[51] demonstrated that in OCP users, procoagulatory increases in fibrinogen and fibrinopeptide A levels are balanced by a compensatory increase in antithrombin III levels. However, in OCP users who smoke cigarettes, there is no corresponding increase in antithrombin III levels, which predisposes these patients to an increased hypercoagulable state.[51] Fruzzetti et al also showed that the increased risk for thrombotic events was primarily estrogen mediated. In their study of coagulation parameters in tobacco smokers and nonsmokers taking oral contraceptives containing 20, 30, or 35 μg EE, Fruzzetti and colleagues[52] found the greatest alteration in smokers and nonsmokers taking the 35 μg dose (Table 2-3). There was only a minimal effect on coagulation parameters in smokers and nonsmokers taking the 20 μg dose. This study suggests that there may be a benefit of using a 20 μg EE OCP to reduce the risk of clinical VTE events, especially among those who smoke.

Opinion on the use of OCPs by women who smoke is divided. The Association of Reproductive Health Professionals (ARHP) states that women <35 years who smoke cigarettes may be advised to use a 20 μg EE OCP and that women >35 years who smoke cigarettes should be advised of the increased risk of adverse vascular events and should not use combination OCPs.[53] One exception to this rule may be the woman >35 years who is a light smoker (<15 cigarettes/day) and insists on using a combination OCP. In light of the minimal effect of smoking on coagulation parameters in women using a 20 μg EE OCP, the ARHP and another consensus panel[54] suggest that women who understand the risks may use a combination or a progestin-only OCP. In contrast, the American College of Obstetricians and Gynecologists (ACOG) states that 'the risk of using OCs is likely to exceed the risk of pregnancy' in female cigarette smokers >35 years.[19] Another consensus panel did not endorse the use of combination OCPs in women >35 years who smoke, regardless of the number of cigarettes smoked.[46]

Former smokers can be considered nonsmokers with regard to OCP use. A 'former smoker' has been defined by one group as someone who has stopped smoking for at least 6 consecutive months;[55] the ARHP definition specifies at least 12 consecutive months.[56] Women who use alternative forms of nicotine (eg, patches, gum) should be managed as tobacco smokers.[53]

Effect of an Inherited Coagulation Disorder and OCP Use

The factor V Leiden mutation is the most common inherited coagulation disorder. It is also the most common genetic cause of thrombosis identified to date, and it accounts for 30% of all VTE events. It is a single-point mutation at codon 506, where adenine is replaced by guanine, and leads to a glutamine substitution for arginine in the factor V protein. The altered factor V protein is rendered resistant to degradation by activated protein C, which results in an increased amount of factor V that stimulates the coagulation cascade by increasing the generation of thrombin. The point mutation is detected by a blood test using the polymerase chain reaction method. The carrier frequency of the factor V Leiden mutation in the United States is 5.27% in whites, 2.21% in Hispanics, 1.25% in Native Americans, 1.23% in African Americans, and 0.45% in Asian Americans.[56] Although these prevalence numbers seem high, especially in whites, the number of people with the mutation who experience a VTE event is low and does not justify mass screening of all patients before prescribing OCPs. In clinical practice, the most important criteria to define who should be screened for the factor V Leiden mutation are a previous VTE event and/or a positive family history of VTE in a first-degree relative.

If a woman is a factor V Leiden mutation carrier, her relative risk of developing a VTE is approximately 6 to 8 times greater than that of the general population, affecting 24 to 40 women/100,000 women annually. If a factor V Leiden mutation carrier uses a low-dose OCP, her RR increases by 30-fold over baseline levels (120 to 150 VTEs/100,000 women annually). Women who are homozygous for the factor V Leiden mutation have the highest RR, with an 80-fold increase in the incidence of VTE, or approximately 320 to 400 cases/100,000 women per year.[57]

Role of Progestins in the Development of VTE Events

Four epidemiologic studies examining OCP use and the risk for VTE events were published in the United Kingdom in 1995 and 1996.[58-61] All four studies (one cohort, three case-control) had adequate sample sizes, and all demonstrated a roughly twofold (1.5- to 2.5-fold) increased risk for VTE events with third-generation progestins (particularly DSG and gestodene) compared with the second-generation progestin LNG. There were insufficient data to draw any conclusions regarding NGM. Although there is no physiologic basis for progestins to increase the risk for VTE events, Rosing et al[62] have advanced a possible explanation for these findings. After studying the effects of various progestins on coagulation factors, they concluded that women taking OCPs with a third-generation progestin like DSG might acquire resistance to activated protein C. This research has been criticized for being a nonrandomized, cross-sectional study with methodological flaws in which blood samples were obtained at different times during the cycle.[63] In contrast to the Rosing study, Schramm and Heinemann[64] found no difference between the effects of second- and third-generation progestins on activated protein C sensitivity.

In response to the four epidemiologic studies, Suissa et al[65] cautioned clinicians not to switch patients based on the studies' findings. They pointed out several possible biases and confounding factors, including the possibility of preferential prescribing of third-generation progestins for women at highest risk and for young women with no pregnancy history, who might be more prone to a thromboembolic event. They also cited the healthy user effect as a confounder. Patients kept on a medication for a long time continue the therapy primarily because they are healthy users without any apparent complications. Therefore, women who have been taking second-generation progestins for a long time have a different number of initial experiences (eg, side effects, complications) with the medication than women who have been taking third-generation progestins for a short time. When Suissa et al reanalyzed the data from the Transnational Study[61] and examined first-time OCP users only, they eliminated the healthy user effect and found no difference between the second- and third-generation progestins. Speroff [66] has suggested another possible confounding factor, noting that women who are heterozygous for the factor V

Leiden mutation and use OCPs have a 30-fold greater RR for and an increased incidence of VTE events than women who are pregnant or use high-dose OCPs. There may have been a disproportionate number of women who were heterozygous for the factor V Leiden mutation in the four epidemiologic studies.

2

After publication of the initial four epidemiologic studies, the British Committee on Safety of Medicines notified all general practitioners in the United Kingdom of the study findings and recommended that women stop using DSG- and gestodene-containing OCPs. In Norway, the Norwegian Medicines Control Agency advised women to reconsider using the one available DSG-containing OCP.[67] This action was followed by a 36% increase in elective abortions in women ≤24 years during the first quarter of 1996. The observed increase in abortions was attributed to women discontinuing their OCPs. In July 1998, the ACOG Committee on Gynecological Practice stated that, based on a possible acquired resistance to activated protein C, the decision to prescribe a DSG formulation should be left to the clinician and the patient.[68]

The potential risk of developing a VTE event was clarified in a recently reported 5-year case-control Danish study.[69] The study examined women 15 to 44 years who had their first DVT or pulmonary embolism between December 1993 and January 1998. A multivariate, matched analysis was performed. The risk of VTE among OCP users was inversely proportional to the duration of use, with ORs of 7, 3.6, and 3.1 for less than 1, 1 to 5, and more than 5 years of OCP use, respectively, compared with women who did not use OCPs. After correction for duration of use and estrogen dose, the RR of a VTE event for users of a third-generation OCP vs a second-generation OCP was 1.3 (1 to 1.8; $P < 0.05$). This increased risk of 33% was determined for OCPs containing DSG or gestodene compared with either LNG or NGM. This study further found that smoking >10 or >20 cigarettes/day, combined with OCP use, increased the risk of a VTE event by 71% and 94%, respectively, compared with OCP use without smoking. The adjusted ORs were 1.7 (95% CI 1.4 to 2.1) and 1.9 (95% CI 1.4 to 2.7), respectively. The negative effect of tobacco smoking on OCP use and the occurrence of a VTE event had not been previously reported.

In summary, all OCPs increase the risk of a VTE event, and the third-generation progestins DSG and gestodene may confer a minimal (33%) increased risk. Further study is needed to clarify the issue. Mass screening for a factor V Leiden mutation is not cost-effective, and screening for the mutation should be limited to individuals with a prior VTE or a history of a VTE event in a first-degree relative.

Effect of OCP Use on the Development of Arterial Thrombosis

The risk of developing a MI or a stroke has been shown to be estrogen dose dependent.[70] The use of low-dose OCPs (≤35 μg EE) does not increase the risk of MI[71] or stroke[72] in nonsmoking, normotensive OCP users.

There is a significant interaction between heavy smoking and OCP use, leading to an increased risk of MI. Croft and Hannaford[73] reviewed data gathered for 20 years (1968 to 1987) in the Royal College of General Practitioners' cohort study of 23,000 OCP users vs age-matched controls. They reported that OCP users who were light smokers had an adjusted RR for MI of 3.5 (95% CI 1.3 to 9.5). OCP users who were heavy smokers had an adjusted RR for MI of 20.8 (95% CI 5.2 to 83.1). As tobacco smoking increases, the RR for an MI increases in OCP users.

In one study, there was an interaction between OCP use and smoking with the development of hemorrhagic, but not ischemic, stroke (P=0.04).[72] The OR for hemorrhagic stroke in women who used low-dose OCPs and smoked was 3.64 vs controls, but the 95% CI of 0.95 to 13.87 is wide and includes 1. In general, stroke is rare among women 15 to 44 years. Low-dose OCPs (≤35 μg EE) do not increase the risk for stroke.

Noncontraceptive Effects of Combination OCPs

Different tissue sites respond differently to the steroids in combination OCPs. At some sites, there is a reduction in the incidence of neoplastic transformation. Such responses comprise some of the noncontraceptive benefits of combination OCPs.

Effect on the Ovaries

After 5 years of combination OCP use, there is a 50% reduction in the incidence of ovarian cancer.[74] This protective effect is seen with low-dose combination OCPs as well as pills with greater amounts of estrogen. After 10 years of combination OCP use, there is an 80% reduction in the incidence of ovarian cancer. The protective effect against ovarian cancer appears to last for 30 years after ingestion of the last OCP.

Effect on the Endometrium

Use of combination OCPs for at least 12 months reduces the incidence of endometrial cancer by 40% (age-adjusted RR=0.6; 95% CI 0.3 to 0.9), and this protective effect persists for at least 15 years after cessation of OCP use.[75] This protection was seen against all three major histologic subtypes of endometrial cancer: adenocarcinoma, adenoacanthoma, and adenosquamous carcinoma.

Effect on the Cervix

Use of combination OCPs has been linked to an increase in cases of carcinoma in situ (CIS) of the cervix, but not cervical cancer.[76] In a population-based, case-controlled study in Costa Rica, women who used OCPs had no increased risk of invasive cervical cancer (RR=0.8; 95% CI 0.5 to 1.3). However, they did have an increased risk of CIS compared with nonusers (RR=1.6; 95% CI 1.2 to 2.2). Further analysis revealed that the increased risk was confined to those who had recently used OCPs and was not elevated in subgroups in which Pap smears were not strongly linked to OCP use. The investigators attributed the increased occurrence of CIS in OCP users to a detection bias because OCP users had more frequent Pap smears.

Effect on the Liver

A large, multinational, hospital-based, case-control World Health Organization (WHO) study found no association between OCP use and liver cancer (RR=0.71, 95% CI 0.4 to 1.2).[77]

Effect on Breast Tissue

In the Canadian National Breast Screening study, there was an inverse association between OCP use and risk of benign breast disease, especially proliferative forms of benign breast disease and benign proliferative epithelial disorders without histologic atypia.[78] The reduction in risk was greater with increasing use for >7 years (RR=0.64; 95% CI 0.47 to 0.87). There was a trend toward increased incidence of benign proliferative epithelial disorders with histologic atypia with >7 years of use, but it was not dose dependent, and the risk included 1 (RR=1.43; 95% CI 0.68 to 3.01).

In a large, population-based, case-control study of US women 35 to 64 years, the risk of breast cancer was not increased in current OCP users (RR=1; 95% CI 0.8 to 1.3) or prior users (RR=0.9; 95% CI 0.8 to 1).[79] Use of OCPs by women with a positive family history of breast cancer or initiation at a young age was not associated with an increased risk of breast cancer. There was also no adverse effect with increasing duration of use or with use of a higher dose of estrogen in current or recent OCP users.

Effect on Acne

Although all combination OCPs can decrease acne by increasing SHBG and decreasing LH production, resulting in decreased circulating levels of testosterone, only two OCPs have obtained FDA approval for the treatment of moderate acne vulgaris. These formulations, Estrostep® Fe and Ortho Tri-Cyclen®, have both demonstrated improvement of acne vs placebo therapy.[80,81]

Diagnosis and Use of Contraception During Perimenopause

Overview

The term perimenopause is used to define an interval of a woman's life prior to actual menopause and ends 12 months after the final menstrual period. Since the timing of the final menstrual period is established retrospectively, it is difficult to prospectively estimate when the perimenopausal period ends. The hallmark of this period is the occurrence of intermittent anovulation that leads to the clinical sign of irregular vaginal bleeding. The vaginal bleeding may have no pattern of frequency, varying from infrequent menses every 12 weeks to daily vaginal bleeding and spotting. The WHO defines the beginning of perimenopause as a break in a woman's regular menstrual cycles but not more than 3 months without a period. When a woman has 3 to 11 months of amenorrhea, she is considered to be in the late perimenopausal period.

The Stages of Reproductive Aging Workshop (STRAW) has clarified terminology and established a staging system for reproductive aging.[82] The perimenopause transition is divided into two stages, the 'early' and the 'late' menopausal transition (Table 2-4). The early menopause transition begins when a woman's regular menstrual cycles become >7 days different from her normal cycle interval (eg, her regular cycles are now every 21 days instead of every 28 days). As a woman's cycle becomes more infrequent, two or more skipped menstrual cycles and at least one interval of amenorrhea of ≥60 days characterize the late menopause transition. Both transitions vary in length and are accompanied by elevated FSH levels. A full year from her final menstrual period, the perimenopausal period is completed and a woman is considered menopausal. Because the duration of the early and late menopause transitions are unpredictable, the entire perimenopause period can last from 2 to 6 years. Because of the inconsistency of this transition,

Table 2-4: The Stages of Reproductive Aging Around the Menopause Period

Stages	**-2**	**-1**
Terminology	Menopausal Transition	
	Early	Late*
	Perimenopause	
Duration of stage	Variable	
Menstrual cycles	Variable cycle length (>7 days difference from normal)	≥2 skipped cycles and an interval of amen (≥60 days)
Endocrine	⇑ FSH	

*Stages most likely to be characterized by vasomotor symptoms.
amen=amenorrhea

it has been said that each woman goes through her own unique perimenopausal period. This intermittent anovulation is similar to the pubertal period where ovulatory cycles are interspersed among anovulatory periods.

Diagnosis of Perimenopause

The use of a menstrual calendar provides an easy, convenient, and reliable method to document the frequency of a woman's period because it will suggest the occurrence of intermittent anovulation. The charting of monophasic basal body temperatures (BBTs) can also demonstrate the

Final Menstrual Period		
+1		+2
Postmenopause		
Early*		Late
(a) 1 yr	(b) 4 yrs	Until demise
amen x 12 mos	None	
	⇑ FSH	

Modified from Soules et al[82]

presence of an anovulatory cycle, but this method is more time-consuming, less convenient, and may not ascertain any additional information. Some individuals will also have difficulty determining if their serial temperatures demonstrate a monophasic or biphasic appearance. A biphasic BBT graph is suggestive of an ovulatory menstrual cycle, while a monophasic BBT graph is associated with an anovulatory menstrual cycle.

The suspicion of anovulation can be further strengthened by the absence of subjective symptoms collectively called 'molimina' before the onset of vaginal bleeding.

Molimina encompasses a group of symptoms, such as breast tenderness, bloating, premenstrual tension, and food cravings, that are synonymous with the fall in progesterone and estradiol levels after ovulation and just before menses.[83] Unfortunately, because of the presence of both ovulatory and anovulatory cycles, laboratory studies are of little value in documenting perimenopause. In a single assessment, the FSH and LH levels may not be elevated because of the intermittent nature of anovulatory cycles. Fluctuations in hormone levels may cause vasomotor symptoms and mood swings during the perimenopausal period. In contrast to menopause, perimenopause is characterized by its relative hyperestrogenism, rather than the constant hypoestrogenic state associated with menopause.

Use of Contraception During the Perimenopause

Because of intermittent ovulatory cycles in perimenopause, women who wish to prevent pregnancy must still use a reliable contraceptive method. The use of combination OCPs provides not only contraception, but also relief from vasomotor symptoms and the irregular vaginal bleeding associated with perimenopause. Women who do not require contraception will still benefit from the improved cycle control and the correction of vasomotor symptoms by OCPs. The use of combination OCPs is not an option for individuals who smoke cigarettes and are >35 years. These women are at increased risk for MI and stroke because of the adverse effect of estrogen on coagulation factors, and are also subject to increased thrombotic risk caused by cigarette smoking. The combined effect of estrogen and cigarette smoking on thrombotic risk appears to be exponentially increased rather than just additive. Because of the dose-dependent effect of estrogen, use of a 20 μg EE OCP formulation is the preferred therapy.[53]

In a randomized, double-blind, placebo-controlled, parallel-group study conducted in Canada, 132 perimenopausal, nonsmoking women with menopausal symptoms were treated with a 20 μg EE OCP for 24 weeks.[84] The 20 μg EE OCP used in this study was Minestrin®, the Canadian brand name for Loestrin® 21 1/20 formulation. The women were between 40 and 55 years. In this study, women treated with OCPs had significantly shortened menstrual cycles ($P < 0.05$), lowered bleeding severity ($P < 0.01$), and improvements in various quality-of-life parameters ($P < 0.01$).

A significant improvement on the 21-day formulation of Loestrin® 21 1/20 has been the addition of three more active pills per pack to form the 24-day formulation Loestrin® 24 Fe. It uses the same steroid formulation as Loestrin® 21 1/20, but has 24 active pills followed by four iron spacer pills. Shortening the pill-free interval from 7 to 4 days is especially important in perimenopausal women, because the absence of circulating contraception levels of EE during the pill-free interval causes FSH levels to rise. This FSH secretion allows the FSH to return to its elevated perimenopausal level. During a 7-day pill-free interval, increased FSH secretion can shorten the follicular phase of the menstrual cycle and can lead to the early selection of a dominant follicle in 5 to 7 days. A dominant follicle is a fluid-filled cyst that contains the oocyte (egg) that is destined to ovulate for that menstrual cycle. Because an oocyte is developing, breakthrough ovulation is possible while using the next pack of OCPs. By shortening the pill-free interval to 4 days, FSH levels are depressed earlier by ingestion of the OCP, and contraceptive levels of EE are reestablished that inhibit FSH release.

In a randomized comparison between Loestrin® 24 Fe and Loestrin® 21 1/20, the 21-day active pill formulation, 938 women were randomized (751 and 187, respectively) for a 6-month study.[25] This study was performed in women 18 to 45 years, and 17% were >35 years. The Pearl Index with Loestrin® 24 Fe was less than the Loestrin® 21 1/20,

21-day product (1.82 vs 2.98, respectively). With Loestrin® 24 Fe, there was also significantly less intracycle bleeding during cycle 6 (0.95 vs 1.63 days, $P=0.005$), and withdrawal bleeding was found to decrease significantly starting as early as cycle 2 and continuing through cycle 6. By the sixth cycle of Loestrin® 24 Fe use, the average length of withdrawal bleeding was more than 1 day less than with the Loestrin® 21 1/20 product (2.66 days vs 3.88 days, respectively, $P<0.001$).

Drug Interactions With Combination OCPs

Certain drugs lead to increased metabolism of OCPs. These agents fall into two classes: anticonvulsants and antimicrobials.

Anticonvulsants

Phenytoin (Dilantin®, Phenytek®), phenobarbital (Solfoton®), and carbamazepine (Carbatrol®, Tegretol®) induce 2-hydroxylation of EE by cytochrome P450IIIA4.[85] Because steroid metabolism is increased, a 35 or 50 μg EE OCP should be used in patients taking these drugs. If a 35 μg EE OCP is used for 9 to 12 weeks without the intervening placebo tablets, the endometrium is more likely to be atrophic and less likely to support the implantation of an embryo in case of a breakthrough ovulation. If these anticonvulsants are discontinued, liver enzymes may stay induced for approximately 4 weeks. During this post-anticonvulsant therapy period, lower-dose OCPs could be used combined with a barrier contraceptive.

The anticonvulsants valproate sodium (valproic acid; Depacon®) and ethosuximide (Zarontin®) do not induce liver enzyme metabolism. There are no indications suggesting an alteration in the prescribing of OCPs with these anticonvulsants.[86,87]

Antimicrobials

Rifampicin (Rifadin®, Rimactane®) also induces 2-hydroxylation of EE by the cytochrome P450IIIA subfamily.[88] If rifampicin is used for a short time, a barrier contraceptive should be added to the OCP therapy. If rifampicin is used for a longer period, adding a 35 μg EE OCP in an extended fashion for 9 to 12 weeks may further help to decrease the likelihood of a contraceptive failure.

2

Use of other antimicrobials, such as penicillin, cephalosporins, and tetracyclines, has not been conclusively linked to more contraceptive failures. Because these antimicrobials are in widespread use, their presence may only be temporally related to the background number of pregnancies (the typical use failure rate) resulting from patient noncompliance with the OCP regimen.

Concept of Dual Methods

Combination OCPs do not protect the user from sexually transmitted diseases (STDs). To decrease the risk of contracting or transmitting a STD, the user should insist that her male partner use a condom. She could alternatively use a female condom.

Brand-name vs Generic OCPs

Many brand-name and generic combination OCPs are available (see Appendix D). Once brand-name products lose their patent protection, generic versions may be developed. Brand-name products are formulations that contain unique components or doses of medication. The Center of Drug Evaluation and Research (CDER) of the FDA must review the product's new drug application, and the manufacturer must obtain approval to produce and market the medication. For generic products to be therapeutically equivalent, they must contain identical amounts of the same active drug ingredients as the brand-name product.[89] They must also be of the same dose, form, route of administration, and strength or concentration.

There can, however, be distinct differences between brand-name and generic products. Even though the generic product must contain the same active ingredients as the branded product, the variability in potency can differ, from

±10% for a branded medication to -20% to +25% of the stated dose for a generic form. The FDA considers two medications to be bioequivalent if the 90% CI limits for the average area under the drug concentration curve (established from dosing studies) of the generic product fall within the range of 80% and 125% of the value of the brand-name medication.[90] The generic product can also differ in shape, color, flavor, presence of preservatives, and/or packaging.[89] The many variations in brand-name and generic OCPs may lead to different blood steroid levels, side effects (eg, uterine bleeding, nausea), poor adherence to the method, or possible unintended conceptions.

Although generic OCP medications contain the same active components as brand-name products, they do not have to be tested for their contraceptive efficacy. Because the FDA does not require clinical trials for generic medication, these products can be released quickly after a brand-name product loses patent protection. The absence of clinical trials makes it difficult to determine the generic medication's true contraceptive efficacy or the occurrence of any unique side effects for a given formulation. Because the developmental cost of a generic medication is less than that for a brand-name product, generic products cost the consumer less. However, the price difference between a brand-name and a generic product may not be enough to justify the occurrence of side effects and/or lost wages from work for physician visits. For example, in March 2005, the average wholesale price of a cycle of a branded product such as Lo/Ovral® was $37.54 vs $30.52 for the generic products Cryselle® and Low-Ogestrel®.[91]

Selecting an OCP

Choosing an OCP can be determined by several criteria. The following section is divided into selecting an OCP based on: a) indication or social situation, b) medical disease state, c) dose of estrogen component, or d) duration of active pills. These recommendations are summarized in Table 2-5.

Indication or Social Situation

Sometimes the choice of an OCP is based upon an indication or social situation that can lead to decreased contraceptive efficacy, such as an established drug interaction with OCPs. Other factors may include a patient's age, her history of cigarette smoking, or body weight. These additional factors can definitely influence the decision for an OCP and sometimes OCPs are contraindicated.

Medications that lead to increase steroid metabolism (eg, anticonvulsants)[86] should use a 35 µg EE OCP in an extended fashion or with a barrier method. Women who are older than 35 years old and do not smoke cigarettes should use a 20 µg EE OCP. Women who are older than 35 years and do smoke cigarettes should not use combination (estrogen- and progestin-containing) OCPs. For women who weigh ≥155 pounds, they should use a 35 µg EE OCP if their pill has 7-day pill-free interval. If their pill has a shorter 4-day pill free interval, the amount of EE in their OCP can be decreased to 20 µg EE daily due to the decreased secretion of FSH during the 4-day vs the traditional 7-day pill-free period. Women using Loestrin® 24 Fe had fewer pregnancies with the 4-day pill-free interval when compared with the 7-day pill-free interval found in Loestrin® Fe 1/20.[25] Both Loestrin® Fe 1/20 and Loestrin® 24 Fe administer 20 µg of EE daily and 28.5% of the entire OCP study group weighed >160 pounds. In this head-to-head trial, the heaviest woman weighed 270 pounds and contraceptive failures (pregnancies) were evenly distributed over the entire range of body weights.

Medical Disease States

Women with hypertension controlled with medication should use a 20 µg EE OCP to minimize their thromboembolic risk. Women using the progestin drospirenone and an ACE inhibitor or angiotensin II receptor antagonist should have their serum potassium monitored to identify

Table 2-5: General Guidelines for Selecting an Oral Contraceptive Pill

Indication or Social Situation

Drug interactions leading to increased metabolism (eg, anticonvulsants)[86]

Age

< 35 years

≥ 35 years

History of cigarette smoking[52]

Age < 35 years

Age ≥ 35 years

Body weight[14]

< 155 lb

≥ 155 lb

Medical Disease States

Hypertension

Diabetes/Insulin resistance

Hirsutism/Acne[80, 81]

Endometriosis

Dysmenorrhea/Premenstrual Syndrome

Dose of Estrogen Component

Early cycle nausea/vomiting

Persistent breakthrough bleeding

Duration of Active Pills

Less frequent menses

Perimenopausal patients, nonsmoker[84]

Age ≥ 35 years, prevent ovarian cysts

20 μg EE OCP*: Loestrin® 24 Fe, YAZ®

20 μg EE OCP**: Graduated estrogen dose OCP, Estrostep® Fe

35 μg EE OCP***: Femcon® Fe, Ortho-Novum® 1/35

2

Recommendation

Use a 35 μg EE OCP*** in an extended fashion or with a barrier method

Use a 20 μg EE OCP* or up to a 35 μg EE OCP***
Use a 20 μg EE OCP*

Use a 20 μg EE OCP*
Do not use a combination OCP

Use a 20 μg EE OCP*
Use a 35 μg EE OCP*** or a 20 μg EE OCP*

Recommendation

Use a 20 μg EE OCP*. Do not use OCP with drospirenone.
Use a 20 μg EE OCP*
Use a 35 μg EE OCP***
Use a 20 μg EE OCP*
Use a 20 μg EE OCP*

Recommendation

Use a 20 μg EE OCP* or **
Use a 35 μg EE OCP***

Recommendation

Use a 20 μg EE OCP* initially, then in an extended use.

Use a 20 μg EE OCP*

OCP=oral contraceptive pill

Table 2-6: Algorithms for Patients Who Miss OCPs

*Algorithm A: Day-Based**

Missed OCPs**	Instructions
Less than 12 hours late	1. Take missed pill immediately. 2. Take next pill at usual time.
More than 12 hours late	Depends on placement in OCP pack. *If pill forgotten in week 1:* 1. Take missed pill immediately. 2. Take next scheduled pill at usual time. 3. If you have had coitus in the last week, consult your doctor for possible emergency contraception (EC). 4. Use a barrier method (eg, condom and/or spermicide) for 7 days. *If pill forgotten in week 2:* 1. Take last missed pill immediately. 2. Leave other missed pills in pack. 3. Take next scheduled pill at usual time. 4. If missed four or more pills, use barrier method (eg, condom and/or spermicide) for 7 days.

*Modified from Korver et al, *Br J Obstet Gynaecol* 1995;102:601-607.

**A missed pill is defined as one that is taken >12 hours late.

the possible complication of resulting hyperkalemia. Unfortunately, when drospirenone is used with the above antihypertensive medications, the risk of hyperkalemia is greater than if either medication is used alone.

2

Algorithm A: Day-Based* *(continued)*

Missed OCPs**	**Instructions**
More than 12 hours late *(continued)*	*If pill forgotten in week 3:* ***Option A:*** 1. Take last missed pill immediately. 2. Leave other missed pills in pack. 3. Take next scheduled pill at usual time. 4. When pack finished, start next pack without a break. 5. Counsel patient on withdrawal uterine bleeding that may occur. ***Option B:*** 1. Stop taking OCPs. 2. Start new pack after 7 pill-free days (count missed-pills days as part of the 7 pill-free days).

(continued on next page)

Hyperkalemia can also develop when drospirenone is used in women concurrently with any medical condition that results in renal insufficiency, hepatic dysfunction, or adrenal insufficiency.

Table 2-6: Algorithms for Patients Who Miss OCPs *(continued)*

Algorithm B: Manufacturer-Based[†]

Type of Missed OCP	Instructions
Placebo pills	1. Throw out those missed.
Other pills	1. Missed one pill in any week? *Take one now. Take the next pill at the usual time.*
	2. Missed two pills in week 1 or 2? *Take two now, two tomorrow. Then take one pill a day until you finish the pack. Use a backup method for 7 days.*
	3. Missed two pills in week 3 or missed three or more pills?
	a. For Day 1 start: *Throw out pack. Start new pack the same day. Use a backup method for 7 days.*
	b. For Sunday start: *Take one pill each day until Sunday. On Sunday throw out pack and start new pack. Use a backup method for 7 days.*

Women with well-controlled diabetes or early insulin resistance should use a 20 μg EE OCP to minimize further small vessel disease.

Women with hirsutism and acne should use 35 μg EE OCP to increase circulating levels of SHBG, which will bind testosterone and decrease the amount of steroid available to bind to receptors in the hair follicle complex and/or within the skin surface.

2

Algorithm C: Absence of Menses

If the patient does not have a withdrawal menses after finishing her OCP pack:

1. If withdrawal menses does not occur within 3 to 5 days after OCPs, obtain a urine or serum pregnancy test.
2. If the pregnancy test is negative, obtain a serum progesterone level to confirm that ovulation has occurred.
3. If the progesterone level is negative for ovulation, restart OCPs in 2 to 4 days.
4. If progesterone level indicates a recent ovulation, wait 9 to 11 days for menses. If no menses occurs after 9 to 11 days, obtain another urine or serum pregnancy test.

†Specific for Wyeth OCPs: Alesse®-28, Lo/Ovral®-28, Ovral®-28, and Triphasil®-28.

Women with endometriosis would have less active disease and dysmenorrhea if their number of menstrual periods per year were reduced. This is due to less menstrual regurgitation of endometrial glands and stromal cells back through their fallopian tubes that can lead to reseeding of the pelvic cavity (and redevelopment of endometriosis) during each menstrual period. Since endometriosis is stimulated by estrogen, a 20 μg EE OCP to minimize estrogen exposure would be preferred. After 3 to 6 OCP cycles of use, women may ingest more active pills to prevent menstrual periods for a specific number of weeks. The use of OCPs in an extended fashion not only decreases the frequency of menses, but it gives the patient's immune system added time to absorb implants of existing endometriosis.

Women with dysmenorrhea and premenstrual syndrome (PMS) should use a 20 μg EE OCP to minimize wide fluctuations in steroid levels that can lead to PMS symptoms. Further use of a shorter pill-free interval and progression onto extended active pill therapy after 3 to 6 OCP cycles further minimizes fluctuations in hormone levels.

Dose of Estrogen Component

In general, a 20 μg EE OCP would be preferable for the initiation of OCPs. This low EE dose will minimize the estrogen side effects of nausea, vomiting, breast tenderness and headaches. An increased amount of EE may be used for women with persistent breakthrough bleeding on 20 μg EE OCPs. A higher dose (35 μg EE) OCP would be indicated for women using the OCP to prevent hirsutism, acne, or the use of other medications that increases sex steroid metabolism.

Duration of Active Pills

The use of a shorter 4-day pill-free interval coupled with 24 days of active pills (Loestrin® 24 Fe) has demonstrated shorter, lighter periods in a comparative trial vs Loestrin® Fe 1/20.[25] Further use of an extended-dose OCP after a period of cyclic use has been shown to decrease breakthrough bleeding in the initial cycles of use.[35] Use of a shorter 4-day pill-free interval would also be preferable in women over 35 years old because of the increased FSH release in the early follicular phase as a woman ages and she shortens the time to develop a dominant follicle. Starting an OCP pack after a 7-day interval increases the likelihood of an unintended ovulation or persistence of the developing follicle with subsequent formation of an ovarian cyst.

Frequently Asked Questions About Combination OCPs

Can you use a multiphasic pill in an extended fashion?

An OCP that changes in estrogen or progestin dose can be used in an extended fashion. As noted above, use of OCPs in an extended fashion should be initiated after the patient has used OCPs for approximately 6 months following the usual protocol of 3 weeks of medication and a subsequent placebo week. After 6 months of OCPs, the endometrium is often uniformly thin, and there is less lining to bleed from. Small alterations in estrogen and/or progestin dose have less overall effect. Some patients who bleed from an atrophic endometrium may benefit from a formulation that changes estrogen dose (eg, Estrostep® Fe). In Estrostep® Fe, the increasing levels of estrogen (20 to 30 to 35 µg) may prevent some vaginal bleeding or spotting caused by increasing atrophy at the level of the endometrial lining. The higher levels of estrogen seem to act similarly to adding exogenous estrogen in other patients who demonstrate atrophic bleeding. Once a woman's endometrium is atrophic, the transition from the 35 µg pills back to the 20 µg pills has not resulted in vaginal bleeding or spotting.

Because OCPs are taken daily, do they build up in your body?

After an OCP is ingested, it dissolves in the stomach and is distributed through the body. The levels of estrogen and progestin do not build up in a woman's body.

I've missed two pills. What should I do?

There are various ways to manage missed OCPs (Table 2-6). One algorithm (Algorithm A) takes into account the position of the missed pill in the OCP pack.[92] It also addresses when extra backup contraceptive precautions are required and for how long. If the bioavailability of the contraceptive steroids is compromised by vomiting or use of an interacting medication, the authors advise modification of the protocol, such as use of dual methods (eg, condoms and/or spermicide) for 7 days or the use of emergency contraception (EC).

In addition to the above general algorithm, OCP manufacturers may have their own product-specific protocols. If a patient misses an OCP, it is advisable to consult the package insert of the OCP in question and follow the manufacturer's instructions. Some manufacturers may have similar instructions for several products (Table 2-6, Algorithm B), despite differences in estrogen dose.

If a patient does not have menstrual bleeding after finishing her OCPs, she may have had a breakthrough ovulation that resulted in a conception or she may have to wait for her circulating level of progesterone to fall to a preovulatory level before she menstruates (Table 2-6, Algorithm C).

I have a history of lactose intolerance, and I've noticed symptoms of diarrhea after taking an OCP. The symptoms don't vary. Could I be lactose intolerant to my pill?

Women who have lactose intolerance should be warned that almost all OCPs contain lactose. One exception is the active pills in the Demulen® formulation. However, the inactive placebo pills in the Demulen® pack do contain lactose. Demulen® is currently available in only one estrogen strength (50 µg EE). Another formulation containing 35 µg EE, Demulen® 1/35, was discontinued in August 2004.

Are multiphasic pills associated with more ovarian cyst formation?

As estrogen levels have decreased in OCPs, ovarian cysts have become more prevalent; however, ovarian cyst formation is not associated to a greater degree with monophasic or multiphasic OCPs.[93] Only higher-dose (>35 µg EE) OCPs have been shown to decrease the formation of ovarian cysts.[94]

Are NET- or LNG-based progestins more androgenic than DSG or NGM?

There are differences in androgenicity among the different progestins, but for the range of progestin doses used in current 20 to 35 μg EE OCPs, there are no clinical differences.[7,8] It is correct to say LNG is more androgenic than NET, DSG, or NGM, but the progestin dose needed to demonstrate a difference in an animal assay is 1,000 times the dose used to inhibit ovulation.[95] At the clinically used doses in OCPs, LNG has no essential androgenic effect. If there is a desire to minimize a progestin's androgenicity, the estrogen-to-progestin ratio in a given estrogen/progestin combination may be increased. For example, the products Ortho-Novum® 1/35, Ortho-Novum® 7/7/7, and Femcon® Fe all contain 35 μg of EE and use 1.0, 0.75 (average amount), and 0.4 mg, respectively, of NET. In comparing these three products, Femcon® Fe would be less androgenic than Ortho Novum® 1/35 and Ortho Novum® 7/7/7.

References

1. The Alan Guttmacher Institute: Facts in Brief: Contraceptive Use. Available at: http://www.guttmacher.org/pubs/fb_contr_use.html. Accessed February 20, 2007.

2. Goldzieher JW, Dozier TS, de la Pena A: Plasma levels and pharmacokinetics of ethynyl estrogens in various populations. II. Mestranol. *Contraception* 1980;21:17-27.

3. Heinen G: The discriminating use of combination and sequential preparations in hormonal inhibition of ovulation. *Contraception* 1971;4:393-400.

4. Kuhnz W, Heuner A, Hümpel M, et al: In vivo conversion of norethisterone and norethisterone acetate to ethinyl estradiol in postmenopausal women. *Contraception* 1997;56:379-385.

4a. Chu MC, Zhang X, Gentzschein, et al: Formation of ethinyl estradiol in women during treatment with norethindrone acetate. *J Clin Endocrinol Metab* 2007;92:2205-2207.

5. US Food and Drug Administration: Yasmin (drospirenone/ethinyl estradiol) Tablets [letter]. Available at: http://www.fda.gov/cder/warn/2003/11730.pdf. Accessed February 26, 2007.

6. Yasmin® package insert. Berlex Laboratories, Montville, NJ, 2004.

7. Breitkopf DM, Rosen MP, Young SL, et al: Efficacy of second versus third generation oral contraceptives in the treatment of hirsutism. *Contraception* 2003;67:349-353.

8. Rosen MP, Breitkopf DM, Nagamani M: A randomized controlled trial of second- versus third-generation oral contraceptives in the treatment of acne vulgaris. *Am J Obstet Gynecol* 2003;188: 1158-1160.

9. Scott JA, Brenner PF, Kletzky OA, et al: Factors affecting pituitary gonadotropin function in users of oral contraceptive steroids. *Am J Obstet Gynecol* 1978;130:817-821.

10. Brenner PF, Mishell DR Jr, Stanczyk FZ, et al: Serum levels of d-norgestrel, luteinizing hormone, follicle-stimulating hormone, estradiol, and progesterone in women during and following ingestion of combination oral contraceptives containing dl-norgestrel. *Am J Obstet Gynecol* 1977;129:133-140.

11. Deligdisch L: Effects of hormone therapy on the endometrium. *Mod Pathol* 1993;6:94-106.

12. Rosenberg MJ, Waugh MS, Meehan TE: Use and misuse of oral contraceptives: risk indicators for poor pill taking and discontinuation. *Contraception* 1995;51:283-288.

13. Baerwald AR, Olatunbosun OA, Pierson RA: Effects of oral contraceptives administered at defined stages of ovarian follicular development. *Fertil Steril* 2006;86:27-35.

14. Holt VL, Cushing-Haugen KL, Daling JR: Body weight and risk of oral contraceptive failure. *Obstet Gynecol* 2002;99(5 pt 1):820-827.

15. Ogden CL, Fryar CD, Carroll MD, et al: Mean body weight, height, and body mass index, United States 1960-2002. Available at: http://www.cdc.gov/nchs/data/ad/ad347.pdf. Accessed February 26, 2007.

16. McNamee B, deVries T: Norethindrone and ethinyl estradiol bioavailability following oral administration of a novel chewable contraceptive tablet in healthy female volunteers. Poster presentation at the annual meeting of the American Association of Pharmaceutical Scientists, Nashville, TN, 2005.

17. Estrostep® Fe Web site. Available at: http://www.estrostep.com. Accessed February 20, 2007.

18. Rosenberg MJ, Waugh MS: Oral contraceptive discontinuation: a prospective evaluation of frequency and reasons. *Am J Obstet Gynecol* 1998;179(3 pt 1):577-582.

19. American College of Obstetricians and Gynecologists: Practice Bulletin. The use of hormonal contraception in women with coexisting medical conditions. July 2000. Available at: http://www.acog.org/publications/educational_bulletins/pb018.cfm. Accessed January 30, 2005.

20. Pratt WF, Bachrach CA: What do women use when they stop using the pill? *Fam Plann Perspect* 1987;19:257-266.

21. Rosenberg M: Weight change with oral contraceptive use and during the menstrual cycle. Results of daily measurements. *Contraception* 1998;58:345-349.

22. Rosenberg MJ, Waugh MS, Stevens CM: Smoking and cycle control among oral contraceptive users. *Am J Obstet Gynecol* 1996; 174:628-632.

23. Killick SR, Fitzgerald C, Davis A: Ovarian activity in women taking an oral contraceptive containing 20 μg ethinyl estradiol and 150 μg desogestrel: effects of low estrogen doses during the hormone-free interval. *Am J Obstet Gynecol* 1998;179:S18-S24.

24. An open-label, multicenter, noncomparative safety and efficacy study of Mircette, a low-dose estrogen-progestin oral contraceptive. The Mircette Study Group. *Am J Obstet Gynecol* 1998;179:S2-S8.

25. Nakajima ST, Archer DF, Ellman H: Efficacy and safety of a new 24-day oral contraceptive regimen of norethindrone acetate 1 mg/ethinyl estradiol 20 micro g (Loestrin 24 Fe). *Contraception* 2007;75:16-22.

26. Yonkers KA, Brown C, Pearlstein TB, et al: Efficacy of a new low-dose oral contraceptive with drospirenone in premenstrual dysphoric disorder. *Obstet Gynecol* 2005;106:492-501.

27. Pearlstein TB, Bachmann GA, Zacur HA, et al: Treatment of premenstrual dysphoric disorder with a new drospirenone-containing oral contraceptive formulation. *Contraception* 2005;72:414-421.

28. Freeman EW, Kroll R, Rapkin A, et al: Evaluation of a unique oral contraceptive in the treatment of premenstrual dysphoric disorder. *J Womens Health Gend Bases Med* 2001;10:561-569.

29. Willis SA, Kuehl TJ, Spiekerman AM, et al: Greater inhibition of the pituitary-ovarian axis in oral contraceptive regimens with a shortened hormone-free interval. *Contraception* 2006;74:100-103.

30. Sulak PJ, Scow RD, Preece C, et al: Hormone withdrawal symptoms in oral contraceptive users. *Obstet Gynecol* 2000;95:261-266.

31. Spona J, Elstein M, Feichtinger W, et al: Shorter pill-free interval in combined oral contraceptives decreases follicular development. *Contraception* 1996;54:71-77.

32. Sullivan H, Furniss H, Spona J, et al: Effect of 21-day and 24-day oral contraceptive regimens containing gestodene (60 microg) and ethinyl estradiol (15 microg) on ovarian activity. *Fertil Steril* 1999;72:115-120.

33. Sulak PJ, Cressman BE, Waldrop E, et al: Extending the duration of active oral contraceptive pills to manage hormone withdrawal symptoms. *Obstet Gynecol* 1997;89:179-183.

34. Sulak PJ, Kuehl TJ, Ortiz M, et al: Acceptance of altering the standard 21-day/7-day oral contraceptive regimen to delay menses and reduce hormone withdrawal symptoms. *Am J Obstet Gynecol* 2002;186:1142-1149.

35. Seasonale® prescribing information. Barr Laboratories, Inc., Pomona, NY, 2003.

36. Alexander NJ, Baker E, Kaptein M, et al: Why consider vaginal drug administration? *Fertil Steril* 2004;82:1-12.

37. Anderson FD, Hait H, Hsiu J, et al: Endometrial microstructure after long-term use of a 91-day extended cycle oral contraceptive regimen. *Contraception* 2005;71:55-59.

38. Anderson FD, Gibbons W, Portman D: Safety and efficacy of an extended-regimen oral contraceptive utilizing continuous low-dose ethinyl estradiol. *Contraception* 2006;73:229-234.

39. Anderson FD, Hait H: A multicenter, randomized study of an extended cycle oral contraceptive. *Contraception* 2003;68: 89-96.

40. Lara-Torre E, Schroeder B: Adolescent compliance and side effects with Quick Start initiation of oral contraceptive pills. *Contraception* 2002;66:81-85.

41. Westhoff C, Kerns J, Morroni C, et al: Quick start: novel oral contraceptive initiation method. *Contraception* 2002;66:141-145.

42. Bracken MB: Oral contraception and congenital malformations in offspring: a review and meta-analysis of the prospective studies. *Obstet Gynecol* 1990;76(3 pt 2):552-557.

43. Schlit AF, Grandjean P, Donnez J, et al: Large increase in plasmatic 11-dehydro-TxB2 levels due to oral contraceptives. *Contraception* 1995;51:53-58.

44. Farmer RD, Preston TD: The risk of venous thromboembolism associated with low oestrogen oral contraceptives. *J Obstet Gynaecol* 1995;15:195-200.

45. US Food and Drug Administration: Talk Paper. Oral contraceptives and risk of blood clots. Available at: http://www.fda.gov/bbs/topics/answers/ans00694.html. Accessed February 20, 2007.

46. Mishell DR Jr, Carr BR, Comp PC, et al: Estrogen doses of oral contraceptives: What are the choices? *Dialogues Contracept* 1996;4:1-12.

47. Gerstman BB, Piper JM, Tomita DK, et al: Oral contraceptive estrogen dose and the risk of deep venous thromboembolic disease. *Am J Epidemiol* 1991;133:32-37.

48. Meade TW, Haines AP, North WR, et al: Haemostatic, lipid, and blood-pressure profiles of women on oral contraceptives containing 50 μg or 30 μg oestrogen. *Lancet* 1977;2:948-951.

49. Speroff L, DeCherney A: Evaluation of a new generation of oral contraceptives. The Advisory Board for the New Progestins. *Obstet Gynecol* 1993;81:1034-1047.

50. Roy S: Effects of smoking on prostacyclin formation and platelet aggregation in users of oral contraceptives. *Am J Obstet Gynecol* 1999;180(6 pt 2):S364-S368.

51. Fruzzetti F: Hemostatic effects of smoking and oral contraceptive use. *Am J Obstet Gynecol* 1999;180(6 pt 2):S369-S374.

52. Fruzzetti F, Ricci C, Fioretti P: Haemostasis profile in smoking and nonsmoking women taking low-dose oral contraceptives. *Contraception* 1994;49:579-592.

53. Association of Reproductive Health Professionals: Clinical Proceedings. Implications of smoking and contraception use. March 1996. Available at: http://www.arhp.org/healthcareproviders/onlinepublications/clinicalproceedings/cpimplicationssmoking/march96.cfm?ID=93. Accessed January 30, 2005.

54. Schiff I, Bell WR, Davis V, et al: Oral contraceptives and smoking, current considerations: recommendations of a consensus panel. *Am J Obstet Gynecol* 1999;180(6 pt 2):S383-S384.

55. Speroff L, Westhoff CL: Smoking and oral contraception. *Dialogues Contracept* 2003;8:4-7.

56. Ridker PM, Miletich JP, Hennekens CH, et al: Ethnic distribution of factor V Leiden in 4047 men and women. Implications for venous thromboembolism screening. *JAMA* 1997;277:1305-1307.

57. Vandenbroucke JP, Koster T, Briët E, et al: Increased risk of venous thrombosis in oral-contraceptive users who are carriers of factor V Leiden mutation. *Lancet* 1994;344:1453-1457.

58. Effect of different progestagens in low oestrogen oral contraceptives on venous thromboembolic disease. World Health Organization Collaborative Study of Cardiovascular Disease and Steroid Hormone Contraception. *Lancet* 1995;346:1582-1588.

59. Jick H, Jick SS, Gurewich V, et al: Risk of idiopathic cardiovascular death and nonfatal venous thromboembolism in women using oral contraceptives with differing progestagen components. *Lancet* 1995;346:1589-1593.

60. Bloemenkamp KW, Rosendaal FR, Helmerhorst FM, et al: Enhancement by factor V Leiden mutation of risk of deep-vein thrombosis associated with oral contraceptives containing a third-generation progestagen. *Lancet* 1995;346:1593-1596.

61. Spitzer WO, Lewis MA, Heinemann LA, et al: Third generation oral contraceptives and risk of venous thromboembolic disorders: an international case-control study. Transnational Research Group on Oral Contraceptives and the Health of Young Women. *BMJ* 1996;312:83-88.

62. Rosing J, Tans G, Nicolaes GA, et al: Oral contraceptives and venous thrombosis: different sensitivities to activated protein C in women using second- and third-generation oral contraceptives. *Br J Haematol* 1997;97:233-238.

63. Winkler UH: Hemostatic effects of third- and second-generation oral contraceptives: absence of a causal mechanism for a difference in risk of venous thromboembolism. *Contraception* 2000; 62(2 suppl):11S-20S.

64. Schramm W, Heinemann LA: Oral contraceptives and venous thromboembolism: acquired APC resistance? *Br J Haematol* 1997; 98:491-492.

65. Suissa S, Blais L, Spitzer WO, et al: First-time users of newer oral contraceptives and the risk of venous thromboembolism. *Contraception* 1997;56:141-146.

66. Speroff L: Oral contraceptives and arterial and venous thrombosis: a clinician's formulation. *Am J Obstet Gynecol* 1998;179: S25-S36.

67. Skjeldestad FE: Increased number of induced abortions in Norway after media coverage of adverse vascular events from the use of third-generation oral contraceptives. *Contraception* 1997;55: 11-14.

68. Weiss G: Risk of venous thromboembolism with third-generation oral contraceptives: a review. *Am J Obstet Gynecol* 1999; 180(2 pt 2):295-301.

69. Lidegaard O, Edström B, Kreiner S: Oral contraceptives and venous thromboembolism. A case-control study. *Contraception* 1998;57:291-301.

70. Meade TW, Greenberg G, Thompson SG: Progestogens and cardiovascular reactions associated with oral contraceptives and a comparison of the safety of 50- and 30-microgram oestrogen preparations. *Br Med J* 1980;280:1157-1161.

71. Sidney S, Petitti DB, Quesenberry CP Jr, et al: Myocardial infarction in users of low-dose oral contraceptives. *Obstet Gynecol* 1996;88:939-944.

72. Petitti DB, Sidney S, Bernstein A, et al: Stroke in users of low-dose oral contraceptives. *N Engl J Med* 1996;335:8-15.

73. Croft P, Hannaford PC: Risk factors for acute myocardial infarction in women: evidence from the Royal College of General Practitioners' oral contraception study. *BMJ* 1989;298:165-168.

74. Ness RB, Grisso JA, Klapper J, et al: Risk of ovarian cancer in relation to estrogen and progestin dose and use characteristics of oral contraceptives. SHARE Study Group. Steroid Hormones and Reproductions. *Am J Epidemiol* 2000;152:233-241.

75. Combination oral contraceptive use and the risk of endometrial cancer. The Cancer and Steroid Hormone Study of the Centers for Disease Control and the National Institute of Child Health and Human Development. *JAMA* 1987;257:796-800.

76. Irwin KL, Rosero-Bixby L, Oberle MW, et al: Oral contraceptives and cervical cancer risk in Costa Rica. Detection bias or causal association? *JAMA* 1988;259:59-64.

77. Combined oral contraceptives and liver cancer. The WHO Collaborative Study of Neoplasia and Steroid Contraceptives. *Int J Cancer* 1989;43:254-259.

78. Rohan TE, Miller AB: A cohort study of oral contraceptive use and risk of benign breast disease. *Int J Cancer* 1999;82:191-196.

79. Marchbanks PA, McDonald JA, Wilson HG, et al: Oral contraceptives and the risk of breast cancer. *N Engl J Med* 2002;346: 2025-2032.

80. Redmond GP, Olson WH, Lippman JS, et al: Norgestimate and ethinyl estradiol in the treatment of acne vulgaris: a randomized, placebo-controlled trial. *Obstet Gynecol* 1997;89:615-622.

81. Boyd RA, Zegarac EA, Posvar EL, et al: Minimal androgenic activity of a new oral contraceptive containing norethindrone acetate and graduated doses of ethinyl estradiol. *Contraception* 2001;63: 71-76.

82. Soules MR, Sherman S, Parrott E, et al: Executive summary: stages of reproductive aging workshop (STRAW). *Fertil Steril* 2001;76:874–878.

83. Magyar DM, Boyers SP, Marshall JR, et al: Regular menstrual cycles and premenstrual molimina as indicators of ovulation. *Obstet Gynecol* 1979;53:411-414.

84. Casper RF, Dodin S, Reid RL, et al: The effect of 20 μg ethinyl estradiol/1 mg norethindrone acetate (Minestrin™), a low-dose oral contraceptive, on vaginal bleeding patterns, hot flushes, and quality of life in symptomatic perimenopausal women. *Menopause* 1997;4:139-147.

85. Ball SE, Forrester LM, Wolf CR, et al: Differences in the cytochrome P-450 isozymes involved in the 2-hydroxylation of oestradiol and 17 a-ethinyloestradiol. Relative activities of rat and human liver enzymes. *Biochem J* 1990;267:221-226.

86. Back DJ, Orme ML: Pharmacokinetic drug interactions with oral contraceptives. *Clin Pharmacokinet* 1990;18:472-484.

87. Kutt H: Interactions between anticonvulsants and other commonly prescribed drugs. *Epilepsia* 1984;25(suppl 2):S118-S131.

88. Combalbert J, Fabre I, Fabre G, et al: Metabolism of cyclosporin A. IV. Purification and identification of the rifampicin-inducible human liver cytochrome P-450 (cyclosporin A oxidase) as a product of P450IIIA gene subfamily. *Drug Metab Dispos* 1989;17:197-207.

89. US Food and Drug Administration: Frequently Asked Questions to CDER. September 2002. Available at: http://www.fda.gov/cder/about/faq. Accessed February 28, 2007.

90. US Food and Drug Administration: Guidance for industry. Bioavailability and Bioequivalence Studies for Orally Administered Drug Products—General Considerations. July 2002. Available at: http://www.fda.gov/cder/guidance/4964dft.pdf. Accessed February 5, 2005.

91. *Red Book Update.* Thomson Healthcare, Inc, Montvale, NJ, vol 24, 2005, pp 32, 50-51.

92. Korver T, Goorissen E, Guillebaud J: The combined oral contraceptive pill: what advice should we give when tablets are missed? *Br J Obstet Gynaecol* 1995;102:601-607.

93. Grimes DA, Godwin AJ, Rubin A, et al: Ovulation and follicular development associated with three low-dose oral contraceptives: a randomized controlled trial. *Obstet Gynecol* 1994;83:29-34.

94. Vessey M, Metcalfe A, Wells C, et al: Ovarian neoplasms, functional ovarian cysts, and oral contraceptives. *Br Med J (Clin Res Ed)* 1987;294:1518-1520.

95. Thorneycroft IH: Update on androgenicity. *Am J Obstet Gynecol* 1999;180:288-294.

Chapter 3

Steroid Contraception: Progestin-only Oral Contraceptive Pills

As their name implies, progestin-only pills (POPs) contain only one steroid, a progestin formulation. They also use a lower dose of medication than that found in combination estrogen/progestin oral contraceptive pills (OCPs). The decreased amount of progestin is responsible for the unique properties of the POP and distinguishes it from combination OCPs.

The primary use of POPs for contraception is in women with conditions in which estrogen is contraindicated or less desirable. These conditions are current thromboembolic disorder (deep vein thrombosis [DVT] or pulmonary embolism), thrombophlebitis, cerebrovascular disease, or coronary occlusion, or a history of or a predisposition to one of these conditions; systemic lupus erythematosus with and without vascular disease; cigarette smoking (in women >35 years); breastfeeding; and history of increased migraine headaches with combination OCPs.

Contraceptive Mechanism and Efficacy

The lower dose of progestin in POPs does not consistently inhibit ovulation. Instead, it prevents conception by acting to develop thick, hostile cervical mucus and to atrophy the endometrium. In one study of 35 users of a POP containing 0.3 mg of norethindrone (NET), 12 women (32%) had follicular and luteal function, while 10 women

(29%) had luteal function consistent with normal ovulation.[1] In total, 63% of women (22/35) had some or normal luteal function while using a 0.3 mg NET formulation.

The quality of the cervical mucus changes within 3 to 4 hours of pill administration;[2] however, because the amount of progestin ingested is small, the effect decreases at 22 hours. At 24 hours from pill ingestion, sperm penetration is not impaired. Women who use POPs for contraception should take their medication at the same time each day to ensure an adequate circulating progestin level to consistently alter the cervical mucus production.

3

The contraceptive failure rate for POPs varies, depending on the clinical indication and compulsiveness of the POP user. Some contraceptive efficacy studies include women who are breastfeeding or >40 years old. These factors are associated with inherent decreased cycle fecundity. In perfect use, the estimated contraceptive failure rate is reported to be 0.3%[3] (see Appendix A). In one study of typical use of POPs by 358 women for up to 150 months (18,125 woman-months of use), three pregnancies occurred.[4] None of the women studied were breastfeeding. The Pearl Index for this group of women was 0.2/100 woman-years. In a study by Vessey et al,[5] the failure rate was higher in younger women (3.1/100 woman-years) compared with women older than 40 years (0.3/100 woman-years).

Proper Use of the POP

The first POP should be taken on the first day of menses, and one pill should be taken daily thereafter. A barrier backup method should be used for the first 7 days of pill administration. If a pill is taken 3 or more hours after the normal ingestion time, a backup method should be used for 2 days. If two or more pills are missed, the next pill should be taken as soon as possible, and a backup method should be used for 7 days. If the patient does not have any vaginal bleeding 4 to 6 weeks later, a pregnancy test should be obtained to rule out an unplanned conception.

POPs can be started immediately after delivery in women who are breastfeeding.[6] They have no adverse effect on breastfeeding as judged by milk volume or infant growth and development.[7,8]

In the United States, NET and norgestrel POPs are available (see Appendix D). The NET POPs contain a dose of 0.35 mg of NET. The norgestrel POP contains 0.075 mg of norgestrel, which is equivalent to 0.0375 mg of levonorgestrel after initial metabolism. In other countries, Femulen® (0.5 mg of ethynodiol diacetate), Microval® (0.03 mg levonorgestrel), and Cerazette® (0.075 mg desogestrel) may be available.

Concept of Dual Methods

The use of POPs for contraception does not protect the user from sexually transmitted diseases (STDs). To decrease the risk of contracting or transmitting a STD, the user should insist that her male partner use a condom. She could alternatively use a female condom.

Side Effects

Because of the unopposed progestin formulation, irregular vaginal bleeding is the primary side effect and the most common reason (47.5%) for POP discontinuation.[4] In addition to vaginal bleeding, POP use leads to an increase in ovarian cyst formation caused by the lack of estrogen-inhibiting follicle-stimulating hormone (FSH) release. In a study by Tayob et al,[9] 38% of POP users (8/21 women) developed a functional cyst, compared with 5% of control women (1/21 women). The maximum diameter of the cysts ranged between 30 and 58 mm.

Breastfeeding Latina women who have a history of gestational diabetes appear to have a threefold increase in developing diabetes mellitus when using POPs.[10] One hypothesis is that the unopposed progestin has a negative effect on insulin metabolism, leading to resistance. Insulin resistance does not occur in women who breastfeed and use a combination OCP.

Drug Interactions With POPs

Similar to combination OCPs, the smaller progestin dose of POPs is susceptible to increased liver metabolism induced by certain anticonvulsants (ie, phenytoin [Dilantin®, Phenytek®], phenobarbital [Solfoton®], carbamazepine [Carbatrol®, Tegretol®]), and the antimicrobial rifampicin [Rifadin®, Rimactane®]. If a patient requires these medications on a chronic basis, a contraceptive option other than a POP should be considered.

Frequently Asked Question About POPs

I currently use 900 mg/day of St. John's wort for depression. I also have migraine headaches that increase in severity when I've used combination OCPs. Can I use a POP for contraception?

St. John's wort is an herb (*Hypericum perforatum*) that is often used as an antidepressant. It can induce increased liver metabolism of steroids and render POPs less effective. The use of POPs for contraception in patients using St. John's wort is not recommended, unless a backup barrier method is also added for further protection.

References

1. Kim-Bjorklund T, Landgren BM, Johannisson E: Morphometric studies of the endometrium, the fallopian tube and the corpus luteum during contraception with the 300 μg norethisterone (NET) minipill. *Contraception* 1991;43:459-474.

2. McCann MF, Potter LS: Progestin-only oral contraception: a comprehensive review. *Contraception* 1994;50:S1-S195.

3. Trussell J: Contraceptive efficacy. In: Hatcher RA, Trussell J, Stewart F, et al: *Contraceptive Technology*, 18th ed. New York, NY, Ardent Media, 2004, p 792.

4. Broome M, Fotherby K: Clinical experience with the progestogen-only pill. *Contraception* 1990;42:489-495.

5. Vessey MP, Lawless M, Yeates D, et al: Progestogen-only oral contraception. Findings in a large prospective study with special reference to effectiveness. *Br J Fam Plann* 1985;10:117-121.

6. Dunson TR, McLaurin VL, Grubb GS, et al: A multicenter clinical trial of progestin-only oral contraceptive in lactating women. *Contraception* 1993;47:23-35.

7. Progestogen-only contraceptives during lactation. I. Infant growth. World Health Organization Task Force for Epidemiological Research on Reproductive Health, Special Programme of Research, Development and Research Training in Human Reproduction. *Contraception* 1994;50:35-53.

8 Progestogen-only contraceptives during lactation. II. Infant development. World Health Organization Task Force for Epidemiological Research on Reproductive Health, Special Programme of Research, Development and Research Training in Human Reproduction. *Contraception* 1994;50:55-68.

9. Tayob Y, Adams J, Jacobs HS, et al: Ultrasound demonstration of increased frequency of functional ovarian cysts in women using progestogen-only oral contraception. *Br J Obstet Gynaecol* 1985;92:1003-1009.

10. Kjos SL, Peters RK, Xiang A, et al: Contraception and the risk of type 2 diabetes mellitus in Latina women with prior gestational diabetes mellitus. *JAMA* 1998;280:533-538.

Chapter 4

Steroid Contraception: The Patch and Vaginal Ring

4

The Contraceptive Patch

Transdermal delivery of contraceptive steroids offers some advantages over orally administered medication. Changing contraceptive patches weekly results in less fluctuation in estrogen and progestin levels than consuming a daily oral medication. Transdermal contraceptive steroids also avoid the first-pass effect through the liver, with less adverse effect on liver parameters. Disadvantages of transdermal delivery include the visibility of the patch and application site reactions.

Product Available in the United States

Ortho Evra® (Ortho-McNeil Pharmaceutical, Inc.) http://www.orthoevra.com

The Ortho Evra® patch is a combination estrogen/progestin transdermal patch that contains 750 µg of ethinyl estradiol (EE) and 6 mg of norelgestromin (the active metabolite of the progestin norgestimate [NGM]) (Figure 4-1). The patch is 4.5 cm square, and it is set to deliver 20 µg of EE and 0.15 mg of norelgestromin/day. By the third day of patch use, hormone levels reach a steady state.

Initiation Methods

Users apply one patch to the lower abdomen or buttocks every 7 days for 3 consecutive weeks. After three consecutive patches, users do not apply a patch for 7 days, and a withdrawal menses occurs.

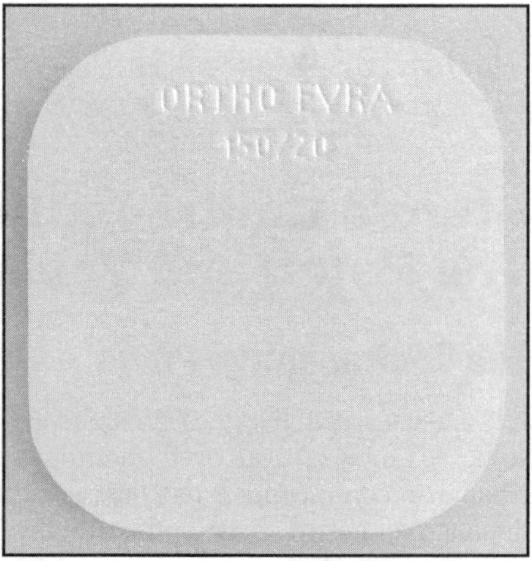

Figure 4-1: The Ortho Evra® patch.

Typical Use

Using one patch/week for three consecutive weeks is associated with approximately a 20% incidence of breakthrough bleeding or spotting. In a comparative study of the Ortho Evra® patch vs Triphasil® oral contraceptive pills (OCPS), there was no significant difference in contraceptive efficacy and cycle control.[1] However, the Ortho Evra®'s contraceptive effect was achieved with a 20 μg EE formulation rather than a 30 μg product that increases to 40 μg EE for 5 days on days 7 to 11 of the pill pack. With respect to overall compliance, patch users were statistically significantly more likely to have perfect compliance than pill users (88.2% and 77.7%, respectively).

Extended Use

Similar to OCPs, the patch can be used for more than 3 consecutive weeks to delay the onset of withdrawal menses. This is an off-label use of the product. In a multicenter study of 200 menstruating women randomly assigned to either a combination transdermal patch in an extended fashion or the usual 3 weekly patch applications, women using the extended protocol had less bleeding than those using the cyclic regimen.[2] The two protocols tested were (1) weekly patch application for 12 weeks followed by 1 patch-free week and 3 weeks of weekly patch application and (2) four consecutive cycles with 3 weekly patch applications followed by 1 patch-free week. In these two protocols, the median time to first bleed was significantly delayed to 54 days in the extended regimen vs 25 days in the cyclic therapy ($P<0.001$). In the final 28-day cycle, women in the extended protocol had 'half as much bleeding' compared with those in the cyclic protocol. There was a similar number of new contraceptive users in the two groups, 43% in the extended protocol and 45% in the cyclic protocol. Women who had prior use of steroid contraceptives had less vaginal bleeding than new contraceptive patients. There was no difference in total vaginal bleeding and spotting days or in patient satisfaction between the two protocols.

Similar to the extension of OCPs, the extended use of patches would be associated with less breakthrough bleeding if a woman has used the patch for at least 6 months before using it in an extended fashion. After 6 months of initial use, a thinner atrophic endometrium will be present, and less breakthrough bleeding should occur.

Contraceptive Mechanism and Efficacy

The patch method works in a similar fashion to combination OCPs, but delivers the steroids transdermally. In a pooled research study of three similar trials, the contraceptive method failure Pearl Index was 0.7 through 13 cycles of patch use (95% confidence interval [CI] 0.31 to 1.1), similar to that for OCPs.[3] This study, however, demonstrated decreased contraceptive efficacy with increased body weight. In 22,160 cycles of use, there were 15 failures (12 method, 3 user), for a method failure rate

Table 4-1: Distribution of 15 Contraceptive Failures With Respect to Body Weight While Using the Ortho Evra® Patch

Body Weight, kg (lb)	Pregnancies	Decile
<52 (<114)	1	1
52 to <55 (<121)	2	2
55 to <63 (<139)	2	3, 4, 5
63 to <69 (<152)	1	6, 7
69 to <74 (<163)	0	8
74 to <80 (<176)	2	9
80 to <90 (<198)	2	10
>90 (>198)	5*	

* $P<0.001$

In a pooled research study of three similar trials encompassing 22,160 cycles of patch use in 3,319 women, the contraceptive method failure Pearl Index was 0.7 through 13 cycles of use, similar to oral contraceptive pills (OCPs). This study, however, demonstrated decreased contraceptive efficacy with increased body weight. Five of the 15 failures occurred in women who weighed >90 kg (>198 lb), who accounted for only 3% of the study population (6% failure rate).

Modified from Zieman et al[3]

of 0.7 (Table 4-1). Five of the 15 failures occurred in women who weighed >90 kg (>198 lb), who accounted for only 3% of the study population. There was a statistically significant increased risk of failure when women weighing >90 kg used the patch (6% failure rate). This higher failure rate may be caused by sequestration of the contraceptive steroids in fat cells, which may decrease circulating serum hormone levels.

This pooled study may have further understated the failure rate of the patch in women weighing >74 kg (163 lb) because the median weight for the study group was approximately 63 kg (139 lb), rather than the national average weight of 74 kg.[4] If a heavier, more representative group of women was studied, there would likely be more conceptions in the 74 to 80 kg and 80 to 90 kg groups.

4

In this pooled data study, four of the five pregnancies in women weighing >90 kg occurred in one study.[5] Of the six pregnancies that occurred in the smaller study, four were in women weighing >90 kg, and one was in a woman who weighed 89.5 kg. The data from this study and the larger pooled data suggest that the Ortho Evra® patch may be less effective in women who weigh >90 kg. This information is listed in the product's package insert. Women who weigh >90 kg and want to use the patch may need to use an additional backup method of contraception.

Circulating Serum Steroid Levels

Although the Ortho Evra® patch is set to deliver 20 µg of EE and 0.15 mg of norelgestromin/day, the circulating steady-state serum levels of both steroids are markedly greater than the 35 µg EE OCP Ortho-Cyclen® (Figure 4-2). Of primary concern is the possibility that transdermal administration of EE leads to higher circulating levels of EE than seen with oral intake, and that this elevated level may lead to an increased risk for a deep vein thrombosis (DVT) or a pulmonary embolism (PE). Collectively, DVT and PE are referred to as venous thromboembolism (VTE). Because of the patch's continuous delivery of steroids, circulating serum levels of EE steadily rise and reach a steady-state level in approximately 3 days. The mean steady-state EE level while wearing the

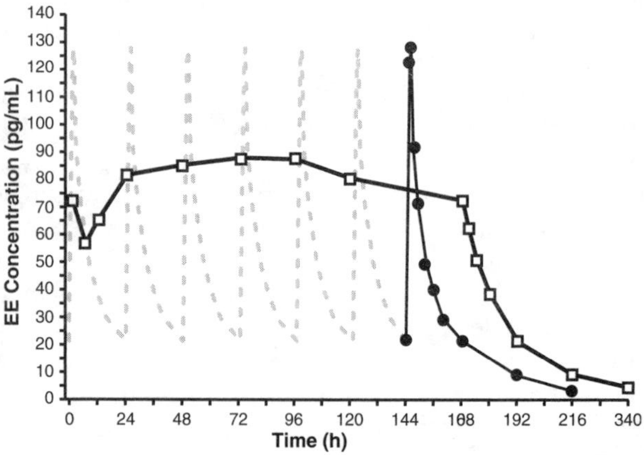

	Ortho Evra®	Ortho-Cyclen®
C_{ss} (pg/mL)	80	49
C_{max} (pg/mL)	97.4	133
AUC_{0-168} (pg·hr/mL)	12,971	8,281

$AUC_{0\text{-}168}$=area under the curve from time 0-168 hours.

C_{max}=maximum concentration

$C_{ss=}$mean steady-state concentration

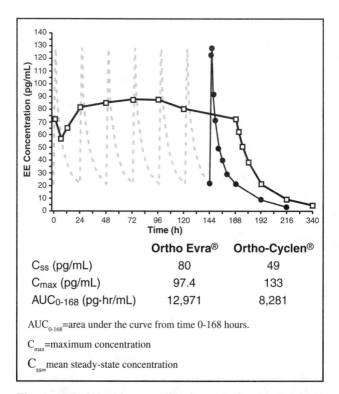

Figure 4-2: Weekly exposure to ethinyl estradiol (EE) from the Ortho Evra® patch and Ortho-Cyclen® pills. Mean serum EE levels from the application of Ortho Evra® (squares) for 2 cycles to the buttocks (cycle 2, week 3) or after ingestion of once-daily Ortho-Cyclen® (filled circles) for 2 cycles (cycle 2, day 21) in healthy female volunteers (n=32). Other Ortho-Cyclen® levels (dotted line, days 15-20, hours 0-144) are estimated from day 21 levels. The mean steady-state EE concentration (C_{ss}) while wearing the Ortho Evra® patch for 2 cycles is 80 pg/mL, which is 62% greater than the 49 pg/mL level with the Ortho-Cyclen® OCP. From Ortho Evra® prescribing information, Ortho-McNeil Pharmaceutical, Raritan, NJ, 2005.

Ortho Evra® patch for 2 cycles is 80 pg/mL, which is 62% greater than the 49 pg/mL level while wearing the Ortho-Cyclen® OCP for the same period of time.[6] Similarly, the area under the curve (AUC) of the steroid concentration vs time for EE is 57% greater for the Ortho Evra® patch vs the Ortho-Cyclen® OCP. In contrast, because of the daily ingestion of an OCP, the maximum concentration (C_{max}) of EE is 37% greater with Ortho-Cyclen® vs Ortho Evra®. This higher maximum level is only transiently elevated and, therefore, the AUC parameter is a more accurate reflection of the greater overall estrogen exposure with Ortho Evra® compared with the 35 μg EE OCP Ortho-Cyclen®.

4

In a comparison of circulating EE levels of Ortho Evra® with a 30 μg EE OCP, Marvelon® (Desogen®), and the 15 μg EE vaginal ring, NuvaRing®, the mean EE level of Ortho Evra® was 63% greater than the 30 μg EE OCP.[7] The average circulating levels of EE in women using the patch, OCP, and ring were 70.9 pg/mL, 43.5 pg/mL, and 21.1 pg/mL, respectively (Table 4-2). These average circulating EE levels were obtained during a 3-week treatment period in women with an average weight of 70.4, 67.4, and 61.2 kg, respectively. These studies and others have consistently found higher inter-subject variability in circulating EE levels compared with women using OCPs. This variability can be attributed to patch placement, the percentage of body fat in the surrounding area of the patch's location, and a patient's body weight. Patches placed on the abdomen had 20% lower circulating EE levels than patches placed on the arm, buttock, and torso.[8] In this study of different patch locations, women had an average weight of 65 kg and no one weighed <50 kg. In women weighing <50 kg, higher circulating levels of EE would be expected than in women weighing 65 to 70 kg.

To determine if increased circulating levels or constant exposure to higher circulating steady-state EE levels leads to more thromboembolic events, results from two epide-

Table 4-2: Average Circulating Level of EE Using the Ortho Evra® Patch, Marvelon® (Desogen®) Oral Contraceptive Pill (OCP), and the NuvaRing® During 21 Days of Use

	Ortho Evra® Patch	Marvelon® (Desogen®) OCP	NuvaRing®
EE per day	20 µg	30 µg	15 µg
EE, average concentration (pg/mL)	70.9	43.5	21.1
Weight (kg)	70.4	67.4	61.2

Prepared from van den Heuvel MW et al[7]

miologic studies have been recently reported.[9,10] The initial study demonstrated a nonsignificant increase in VTE with the Ortho Evra® patch (52.8/100,000 woman-years) compared with the 35 µg EE OCP with NGM Ortho-Cyclen® and Ortho Tri-Cyclen® (41.8/100,000 woman-years).[9] This study appears to confirm that the patch has similar risks to a 35 µg EE OCP and, although set to deliver 20 µg of EE/day, should not be classified with other OCPs containing <35 µg of EE. The interim analysis results from the second study, however, revealed a possible twofold increased risk of VTE with Ortho Evra® compared with a NGM-containing OCP with 35 µg of EE.[10] If this result is confirmed, the increased circulating levels of EE seen with use of Ortho Evra® may be more detrimental than low-dose OCPs containing ≤35 µg of EE.

In light of the above findings, women at increased risk for VTE should be aware of the possible effects of increased circulating steady-state levels of EE. At-risk individuals may include women who smoke cigarettes and those weighing <50 kg (<110 lb). This low-weight advisory should be considered since we have less information on circulating levels of EE in thinner subjects. In women at higher risk for thromboembolism and who have demonstrated prior poor compliance with OCPs, the use of lower dose (<35 μg of EE) extended OCP regimens (consuming active OCPs for 6 to 9 weeks) may be more helpful than using OCPs in the standard 3 weeks of active medication followed by a pill-free week. In women with a history of inconsistent OCP consumption who used the patch to increase method compliance, the use of extended-dose OCPs minimizes the effect of intermittently missing an OCP. Alternatively, use of an OCP with a shorter pill-free interval like Loestrin® 24 Fe (24 days of active pills and 4 days of iron placebo pills) or YAZ® (24 days of active pills and 4 days of inert placebo pills) will decrease the chance of an escape ovulation and suppress rising levels of FSH earlier than the usual 21-day OCPs. In some women, use of a different contraceptive method may be more appropriate than using the current Ortho Evra® patch formulation.

Frequently Asked Questions

How do I remove and prevent lint from accumulating on the edges of the patch?

After removing the patch, residual lint may be removed by applying baby oil or an orange oil-based solvent to the skin. Orange oil is derived from the fruit's peel and acts as a natural solvent. It is commercially available in a variety of strengths and sold under a number of different brand names. Applying a light dusting of baby powder to the patch edges will also decrease the amount of lint that attaches to the patch edge/skin interface.

Can I use the patch method if I have a latex allergy?

Patients with latex allergy can use the patch method.

Can I wear the patch under water?

Women can wear the patch under water while swimming or bathing.

If the patch partially or completely detaches, what can I do?

A new patch should be applied after either partial or complete detachment. Reimbursement for replacement patches (up to $12.00) can be obtained from the manufacturer. Replacement patches can be obtained from a local pharmacy.

Can the patch discolor my skin, or can I develop an allergic reaction?

Some individuals may develop skin discoloration or a local allergic reaction. Because patches must deliver medication through a keratinized surface, a permeation enhancer, often alcohol, must be used to overcome this barrier. Some women may become sensitive to the permeation enhancer within the patch.

Are patches that are advertised on the Internet safe?

Not all pharmacies selling medication via the Internet are reputable. The US Food and Drug Administration (FDA) recently closed four foreign Internet sites selling counterfeit contraceptive patches that contained no active contraceptive. These patches were packaged loosely, without labeling information such as lot numbers or expiration dates. The FDA has posted photographs of the fake patches on its Web site at http://www.fda.gov/bbs/topics/news/photos/contraceptive/counterfeit.html. Further information may also be obtained from the Ortho-McNeil Customer Care Center by calling its toll-free telephone number, 1-800-682-6532.

The Contraceptive Ring

Overview

Use of the vagina for the delivery of contraceptive steroids has some distinct advantages over oral and transdermal routes. Unlike oral medication, contraceptive steroids absorbed from the middle and upper third of the vagina drain into veins that contribute directly to the inferior vena cava, bypassing the hepatic portal system. The absence of the hepatic first-pass effect leads to less disruption of lipoproteins and less alteration of hepatic function. The extensive vascular connections between the vagina and the uterus allow steroids absorbed from the vagina to be concentrated in the uterus, leading to a 'first uterine pass' effect. This allows for the use of lower doses of medication and potentially less frequent administration. Vaginally administered medication causes less nausea and gastrointestinal (GI) disturbance than orally administered medication. Vaginal medication is also less susceptible to inadequate absorption when diarrhea is present. In a small study, OCPs were given vaginally, with inhibition of ovulation and less resulting nausea.[11]

In contrast to the transdermal route, there is no keratinized surface in the vagina acting as a barrier to the delivery of medication. The vagina has four distinct layers: a nonsecretory stratified squamous epithelium, a lamina propria or tunica, muscle fibers, and an areolar connective tissue layer with blood vessels.[12] There are no fat (adipose) cells, glands, or hair follicles in the vagina. The absence of a keratinized surface allows for easier absorption of medication, and the absence of adipose tissue prevents the sequestration of steroids, which is one possible reason for lower circulating steroid levels with transdermal medication.

In the case of the vaginal ring for contraception, steady-state hormone levels are easily achieved after insertion because they are less dependent on patient compliance and daily or weekly administration of medication than OCPs or the transdermal patch. One drawback to the vaginal ring is the difficulty in getting young patients to initiate therapy. Many younger women are unwilling to insert a ring into their vagina and leave it in place for 3 weeks.

Product Available in the United States

NuvaRing® (Organon USA, Inc.)
http://www.nuvaring.com
Toll-free telephone number: 1-877-NuvaRing (1-877-688-2746)

The NuvaRing® is a combination estrogen/progestin flexible vaginal ring that releases 15 mg of EE and 0.120 mg of etonogestrel per day (Figure 4-3). Etonogestrel is the active form of the progestin desogestrel (DSG). The ring is made of an ethylene vinyl acetate and is 2 inches (5.4 cm) in diameter and 1/8-inch (4 mm) thick. It is inserted into the vagina, left in place for 3 weeks, and then removed for 1 week. On completion of this time, a new ring is inserted.

Initiation Methods

The user should insert the vaginal ring within the first 5 days of her menstrual period. The ring may be inserted at any time during the menstrual cycle if the user is certain she is not pregnant. Women initiating the use of the NuvaRing® should use a backup method of contraception for 7 days.

Typical Use

The NuvaRing® should not be removed during coitus. In the first cycle of use, approximately 5% to 6% of women report irregular bleeding, which is a lower rate than that associated with OCP use.[13,14] Absence of fluctuation in contraceptive steroid levels associated with patient noncompliance may account for the difference. Withdrawal bleeding occurred in almost all cycles of use; withdrawal bleeding was absent in 0.6% to 2.1% of cycles over cycles 1 to 13

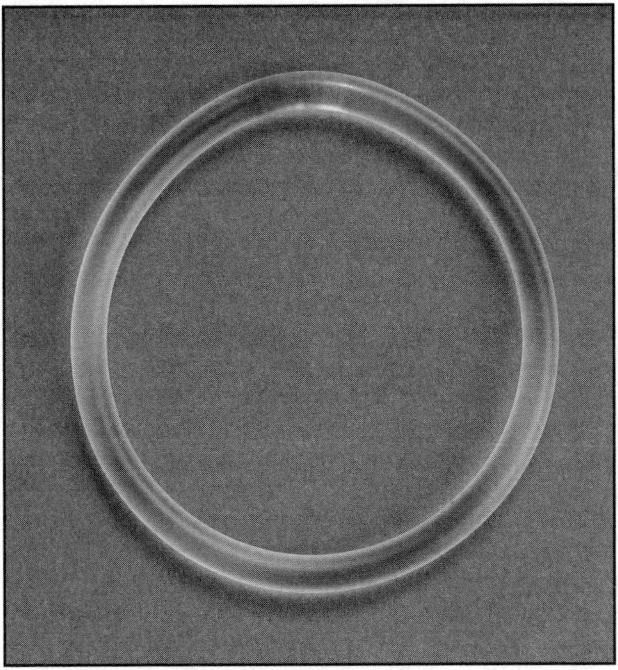

Figure 4-3: The NuvaRing®.

of use.[13] Duration of bleeding over cycles 1 to 13 ranged from 4.7 to 5.3 days (standard deviation=1.7 to 2.5 days). In 5.4% to 7.7% of cycles, withdrawal bleeding started before removal of the ring. In 2.8% to 5.4% of cycles, this bleeding was restricted to vaginal spotting. Women who were switching from combined or progestin-only OCP use reported less early withdrawal bleeding (3.7% to 6%) than new starters of the vaginal ring (7.1% to 12.4%). In 20.4% to 27.3% of cycles, withdrawal bleeding continued beyond the 7-day ring-free interval, but this was confined to vaginal spotting in 16.5% to 21.4% of cycles. After completion of 13 cycles of NuvaRing® use, 91.9% of women reported normal menstruation by the fourth week following removal of the last ring.

Extended Use

The same NuvaRing® can be used for a month—28 to 31 days—changing the ring on the first day of each month. This may help foster increased patient compliance with the product. Using the ring for this extra time, rather than just 21 days, has not been associated with more contraceptive failures. In one study, a single ring suppressed ovulation for 35 days.[15] This additional suppression may be helpful if a woman forgets to remove her ring after 21 days. In an effort to prevent withdrawal vaginal bleeding, the ring could be replaced each month without a week-long removal interval. This therapy could be continued for an extended period (2 to 4 months), or until bleeding from endometrial atrophy occurs. Use of the NuvaRing® in this fashion is similar to the use of extended-dose OCPs and is off-label.

Contraceptive Mechanism and Efficacy

The NuvaRing®, similar to OCPs, inhibits ovulation.[15] The Pearl Index for the NuvaRing® was 0.65/100 woman-years in all first-year users (95% CI 0.24 to 1.41).[8] The typical use failure rate has not been firmly established, but it is estimated to be similar to that of OCPs, at 8/100 woman-years. It is thought that the typical-use failure rate should be lower in ring users than in OCP users because of easier compliance, but women must still remember to remove the old ring and insert a new one at regular intervals.

Side Effects

In a large, multicenter, multinational study involving 2,322 women and 22,298 cycles of experience, the three most common side effects that were at least possibly treatment related during the 1-year study period were headache (5.8%), vaginitis (5.6%), and leukorrhea (4.8%). Device-related adverse events, including foreign-body sensation, coital problems, and/or expulsion, were the next most common (4.4%). Estrogen-related side effects of nausea (3.2%), breast tenderness (2.6%), and acne (2%) were relatively uncommon. This information represents pooled data from two similarly designed studies. One was conducted in 48 centers in the United States and Canada, and the other encompassed the experience in 52 European centers previously reported by Roumen and colleagues.[13]

Frequently Asked Questions

If I have vaginal bleeding while using the NuvaRing®, can I use a tampon?

A tampon can be used with the NuvaRing®. Some early vaginal bleeding and spotting may occur before the 21st day of use. Vaginal withdrawal bleeding may also continue beyond the 7-day ring-free interval.

If I have a vaginal infection and I'm using vaginally administered medication, do I need to remove the NuvaRing®?

The NuvaRing® does not have to be removed when other vaginal medications are used concurrently. As long as the NuvaRing® is in contact with the vaginal walls, medication will be absorbed into the vagina.

Is it uncomfortable to keep the NuvaRing® in the vagina? Does it hurt?

In the upper 75% of the vagina, the nerve supply is primarily autonomic nerve fibers, which are not sensitive to pain or temperature. This allows a vaginal ring or other product (eg, contraceptive sponge, suppository, tampon) to be placed in the vagina without discomfort. In a survey of NuvaRing® users (N=2,128), 83% of women stated they could not feel the ring during intercourse, while 13% and 5% of women stated they occasionally or frequently felt the ring during coitus, respectively.[14]

Will my partner feel the NuvaRing® during sexual intercourse?

In a survey of women using the NuvaRing® (N=2,129), 68% of partners could not feel it during coitus. Of the remaining partners, 22% occasionally and 10% said they frequently felt the ring during intercourse. When ring users were asked if their partner objected to the ring (N=2,133), 91% did not object, 5% occasionally objected, and 5% frequently objected.[14]

If I want to remove the NuvaRing®, for how long can it be removed without loss of efficacy?

The NuvaRing® can be removed for 3 hours without loss of efficacy.

I'm worried that the NuvaRing® will 'get lost up there.' Can that happen?

NuvaRing® users may want to verify that the ring is still in place by intermittently checking for it high in the vagina. A short, concise review of the anatomy of the vagina, specifically mentioning to the patient that the vagina is a closed space, will help address this question. Further instructing the patient on the insertion and removal of the ring and having the patient demonstrate these steps will help to avoid incorrect placement and difficult removal. Occasionally, a patient has unknowingly spontaneously expelled a NuvaRing®, and it cannot be found. It is suggested that women using the NuvaRing® have two rings available, in case the first is lost.

References

1. Audet MC, Moreau M, Koltun WD, et al: Evaluation of contraceptive efficacy and cycle control of a transdermal contraceptive patch vs an oral contraceptive: a randomized controlled trial. *JAMA* 2001;285:2347-2354.

2. Stewart F, Laguardia KD, Kaunitz A, et al: Reducing menstrual bleeding with extended use of transdermal norelgestromin/

ethinyl estradiol: a randomized clinical trial. Available at: http://www.contemporaryobgyn.net/obgyn/article/articleDetail.jsp?id=125959. Accessed February 27, 2007.

3. Zieman M, Guillebaud J, Weisberg E, et al: Contraceptive efficacy and cycle control with the Ortho Evra/Evra transdermal system: the analysis of pooled data. *Fertil Steril* 2002;77: S13-S18.

4. Ogden CL, Fryar CD, Carroll MD, et al: Mean body weight, height, and body mass index, United States 1960-2002. Available at: http://www.cdc.gov/nchs/data/ad/ad347.pdf. Accessed February 27, 2007.

5. Smallwood GH, Meador ML, Lenihan JP, et al: Efficacy and safety of a transdermal contraceptive system. *Obstet Gynecol* 2001; 98:799-805.

6. Ortho Evra® package insert. Ortho-McNeil Pharmaceutical, Inc., Raritan, NJ, 2005.

7. van den Heuvel MW, van Bragt AJM, Alnabawy AKM, et al: Comparison of ethinylestradiol pharmacokinetics in three hormonal contraceptive formulations: the vaginal ring, the transdermal patch and an oral contraceptive. *Contraception* 2005;72: 168-174.

8. Abrams LS, Skee DM, Natarajan J, et al: Pharmacokinetics of a contraceptive patch (Evra/Ortho Evra) containing norelgestromin and ethinyloestradiol at four application sites. *Br J Clin Pharmacol* 2002;53:141-146.

9. Jick SS, Kaye JA, Russmann S, et al: Risk of nonfatal venous thromboembolism in women using a contraceptive transdermal patch and oral contraceptives containing norgestimate and 35 μg of ethinyl estradiol. *Contraception* 2006;73:223-228.

10. Ortho Evra® Web site (http://www.orthoevra.com).

11. Coutinho EM, Coutinho EJ, Goncalves MTR, et al: Ovulation suppression in women following vaginal administration of oral contraceptive tablets. *Fertil Steril* 1982;38:380-381.

12. Alexander NJ, Baker E, Kaptein M, et al: Why consider vaginal drug administration? *Fertil Steril* 2004;82:1-12.

13. Roumen FJ, Apter D, Mulders TM, et al: Efficacy, tolerability and acceptability of a novel contraceptive vaginal ring releasing etonogestrel and ethinyl oestradiol. *Hum Reprod* 2001;16: 469-475.

14. Dieben TO, Roumen FJ, Apter D: Efficacy, cycle control, and user acceptability of a novel combined contraceptive vaginal ring. *Obstet Gynecol* 2002;100:585-593.

15. Mulders TM, Dieben TO: Use of the novel combined contraceptive vaginal ring NuvaRing for ovulation inhibition. *Fertil Steril* 2001;75:865-870.

Chapter 5

Steroid Contraception: Injections and Implants

5

Steroid Injections

Product Available in the United States

Depot-medroxyprogesterone acetate (DMPA)
Depo-Provera® Contraceptive Injection
(Pfizer Pharmaceuticals, Inc.)
http://www.depo-provera.com
Toll-free telephone number:
1-866-554-DEPO
(1-866-554-3376)

Depot-medroxyprogesterone acetate (DMPA) is a progestin that has contraceptive action when administered at a dose of 150 mg intramuscularly (IM) every 3 months or 13 weeks.[1] The US Food and Drug Administration (FDA) approved Depo-Provera® use for contraception in 1992, after a World Health Organization (WHO) study found that there was only a slight or no increase in the risk for breast cancer,[2] an adverse finding that was previously reported in beagle dogs.[3] At a dose of 150 mg IM, the progestin increases in concentration for approximately 3 weeks to a level of 1 to 7 ng/mL. The medication becomes undetectable (<0.1 ng/mL) between 120 and 200 days after injection.[1] Because the medication is given parenterally, compliance is optimal if the patient returns for her injections. This preparation is ideal for patients with contraindications to estrogen-containing contraceptives.

Contraceptive Mechanism and Efficacy

The reported typical failure rate for DMPA is 0.3 pregnancy at 1 year of use (see Appendix A).[1]

The mechanisms of action for this progestin medication include thickening of the cervical mucus, atrophy of the endometrium, and inhibition of ovulation.

Proper Use

Depo-Provera® should be administered to nonpregnant women in the following manner:[1]

1. Depo-Provera® can be administered in the early follicular phase of the menstrual cycle or the postpartum period. If given after menses begins, the medication should be given only during the first 5 days of the menstrual cycle. If given during the postpartum period, Depo-Provera® can be administered in the first 5 days postpartum if not breastfeeding. If the patient is breastfeeding, then Depo-Provera® should be given in the sixth postpartum week.
2. Depo-Provera® is given IM into the gluteal or deltoid muscle.
3. If more than 13 weeks elapse between injections, the health-care provider must determine that the patient is not pregnant before giving the next Depo-Provera® injection.

Concept of Dual Methods

The Depo-Provera® injection does not protect the user from sexually transmitted diseases (STDs). To decrease the risk of contracting or transmitting a STD, the user should insist that her male partner use a condom.

Side Effects

A prospective research study by Berenson et al[4] examining the effect of 2 years of DMPA use on bone mineral density (BMD) measurements of the lumbar spine reported a BMD decrease of 5.74% (95% confidence interval [CI]

-7.90 to -3.57) in 33 DMPA users. There was a -5.94% change (95% CI -7.98 to -3.90) in BMD between DMPA users and 44 control women ($P<0.05$). The study also compared DMPA to two types of oral contraceptive pills (OCPs), one containing 35 μg of ethinyl estradiol (EE) and 1 mg of norethindrone (NET), and the other containing 30 μg of EE and 0.15 mg of desogestrel (DSG). There were significant ($P<0.05$) decreases in BMD among all users, with a 5.27% decrease in the 25 NET users (95% CI -7.61 to -2.93) and a 4.43% decrease in the 42 DSG users (95% CI -6.49 to -2.37). There was no significant difference between the OCPs. This study was performed in adult women 18 to 33 years who self-selected their method of contraception and were within 36% of ideal body weight for height. Similar findings demonstrating changes in adult BMD at the spine, total hip, and femoral neck for 5 years of DMPA use and 2 years post-use are listed in the Depo-Provera® package insert (Table 5-1).[1]

There seem to be similar findings of decreased BMD in DMPA users <18 years compared with controls. In a study of 370 adolescents 12 to 18 years who self-selected DMPA or OCPs, there was a significant 1.4% decrease in BMD at the lumbar spine in DMPA users compared with a 2.8% increase in the OCP users and a 3.8% increase in controls ($P<0.001$).[5] There was also a 2.2% decrease in BMD in the femoral neck of the hip in the DMPA group compared with increases of 0.3% and 2.3% in the OCP and control groups, respectively ($P<0.001$). In a smaller 2-year longitudinal study, Lara-Torre et al[6] demonstrated a -6.81% change in BMD at the lumbar spine after 24 months of self-selected DMPA use (N=21) compared with controls (N=6).[6] Loss of BMD in the adolescent years may be particularly important because BMD accrues exponentially between the ages of 11 and 14 years, followed by a plateau by age 19.[7] Any alteration in adolescent bone mineralization may have a long-term effect on peak BMD and/or the future occurrence of osteoporosis.

Table 5-1: Mean Percent Change From Baseline in Bone Mineral Density (BMD) in Adults by Skeletal Site and Cohort*

Time in Study	Spine	
	Depo-Provera®	*Control*
5 years	N=33 -5.38%	N=105 0.43%
7 years	N=12 -3.13%	N=60 0.53%

* The treatment group consisted of women who received Depo-Provera® for 5 years and were then followed for 2 years post-use. The control group consisted of women who did not use hormonal contraception and were followed for 7 years.

Pregnancy and lactation are associated with short-term BMD changes.[8,9] In a study of 16 women, there was a -4.6% change in lumbar spine BMD shortly after delivery.[8] Losses from pregnancy and lactation return to baseline after delivery and weaning.

Because of the recent reports of BMD loss while using DMPA, the FDA has added new warning information to the Depo-Provera® package insert.[1] The FDA recommendations for adult DMPA users are as follows:

1. Depo-Provera® should be used beyond 2 years only if other birth control methods are inadequate.
2. If Depo-Provera® is used beyond 2 years, a BMD measurement should be obtained.
3. Although there are no studies addressing the effectiveness of calcium and vitamin D therapy, women should have adequate calcium and vitamin D intake.

Total Hip		Femoral Neck	
Depo-Provera®	***Control***	***Depo-Provera®***	***Control***
N=21	N=65	N=34	N=106
-5.16	0.19%	-6.21	-0.27%
N=7	N=39	N=13	N=63
-1.34%	0.94%	-5.38%	-0.11%

From Depo-Provera® contraceptive injection package insert. Pfizer Pharmaceuticals, Inc., New York, NY, 2004.

The FDA recommendations for adolescent DMPA users are the same as those for adults, with the addition that, in adolescents, the interpretation of BMD studies should take into account the patient's age and skeletal maturity.

Women at high risk for developing osteoporosis should consider an alternative contraceptive method when the risk exceeds the contraceptive benefit of DMPA. High-risk women are those with (1) metabolic bone disease, (2) anorexia nervosa, (3) a family history of osteoporosis, (4) chronic alcohol use, (5) chronic tobacco use, and (6) chronic use of medication that can reduce bone mass (eg, corticosteroids, anticonvulsants).

One prominent side effect in patients using DMPA has been an increasing incidence (38% to 46% over 6 months) of progressive weight gain.[10,11] In one study of 53 adolescent females who used DMPA, the average weight gain was 6 kg (13.2 lb) at 11 months of use and 9 kg (19.8 lb) at 17 months.[11] A large, multicenter study of 3,905 women using DMPA for 1 to 6 years documented average increases in weight of 5.4, 8.1, 13.8, and 16.5 lb after 1, 2, 4, and 6 years of DMPA use, respectively.[1,12] Amatayakul et al[13] investigated the mechanism for the apparent weight gain with DMPA use and found an increase in body fat deposition by anthropometric measurements and not by anabolism or fluid retention. DMPA may stimulate appetite, leading to increased food intake and weight.

Because of DMPA's progestin effect, many women will have amenorrhea (46% at 3 months and 58% at 12 months) or some spotting or irregular vaginal bleeding (46% at 3 months and 40% at 12 months).[10] DMPA use can also result in thinning of the vaginal epithelium and increased susceptibility to the human immunodeficiency virus (HIV)[14] and bacterial colonization.

After discontinuation of DMPA, the return to regular menstrual cycles occurs in approximately 6 months. Clearance is slower in heavier women.[15] In a study to determine the return to ovulatory cycles, the average time to ovulation as documented by weekly serum progesterone measurements was 5.5 months after a minimum of 1 year of DMPA therapy.[16] There was no correlation between the duration of DMPA use and the return to ovulatory cycles.

Frequently Asked Question

How long should I use Depo-Provera®?

For adult women ≥18 years, the decision to continue Depo-Provera® use should be reevaluated after 2 years. Women should continue Depo-Provera® therapy beyond 2 years only if other birth control methods are inadequate. If a woman continues to use Depo-Provera®, a BMD measurement should be obtained. If the user is at increased risk for decreased BMD, then another method should be considered. Women who continue DMPA use should adopt a weight-bearing exercise routine and a calcium-rich diet.

The continued use of DMPA should be balanced against the risk of an unintended pregnancy and its negative effect on BMD.

DMPA users <18 years should consider an alternative contraceptive measure to avoid possible suppression of the attainment of peak BMD and the unknown long-term effects of DMPA use on general bone health.

Recalled Product

Lunelle™

Lunelle™ was a combination progestin/estrogen injectable contraceptive medication formulated for monthly IM injection. The components were 25 mg medroxyprogesterone acetate (MPA) and 5 mg estradiol cypionate formulated in a 0.5 mL suspension in a prefilled syringe. The dosing schedule for this medication was every 28 ± 5 days. The FDA approved Lunelle™ for use in October 2000; however, the medication is no longer available in the United States. The manufacturer, Pharmacia Corporation, voluntarily recalled Lunelle™ in October 2002 because of a lack of assurance of full potency and a possible risk of contraceptive failure.

In light of the concern about possible decreased BMD with DMPA, similar anxiety may be warranted for Lunelle™ users despite the presence of estradiol cypionate.

Because of the report of decreased potency and a possible adverse effect on BMD, Lunelle™ may not be reintroduced into the US pharmaceutical market.

Steroid Implants

Implanon™

Organon International
http://www.organon.com
Toll-free telephone number:
1-877-IMPLANON (1-877-467-5266)

Implanon™ is a progestin-based, single-rod contraceptive medication formulated for 3 years of continuous use.

The implant is 4 cm long and 2 mm in diameter. It consists of a central core that contains 68 mg of etonogestrel (3-ketodesogestrel) encased by a membrane of ethylene vinyl acetate copolymer. The etonogestrel is released initially at a rate of 60 μg/day in weeks 5 to 6 of use and decreases to 35 to 45 μg/day at the end of 1 year. The released amount of etonogestrel further decreases to 30 to 40 and 25 to 30 μg/day at 2 and 3 years of use, respectively.[17] The implant is placed in the subcutaneous tissue of the upper arm using a disposable, preloaded inserter.

Implanon™ functions similarly to other progestin-based contraceptives, by creating hostile, thick, cervical mucus and atrophy of the endometrium. There appears to be greater inhibition of ovulation by Implanon™ compared with the original Norplant® implant system. As stated in the package insert, approximately 20% of Implanon™ users had amenorrhea.[17] Implanon™ must still be removed after all the progestin is released, but removal appears to be less difficult than with Norplant®. The Implanon™ copolymer outer membrane may not react with the surrounding tissue as much as Norplant® does, leading to less fibrosis. The shelf life of Implanon™ is 5 years.

On July 18, 2006,the FDA approved the use of Implanon™ in the United States. The manufacturer, Organon, has organized proctored training sessions to instruct practitioners on the proper insertion and removal of the Implanon™ contraceptive rod. The effectiveness of Implanon™ has not been established in women who weigh >130% of their ideal body weight because prior studies excluded women in this weight category.[17] Since circulating etonogestrel levels are inversely related to body weight and decrease over time, practitioners should use Implanon™ with caution in women weighing >130% of their ideal body weight. In addition, women who have other factors that might decrease their etonogestrel levels, such as hepatic enzyme inducers, should also use the Implanon™ contraceptive rod with increased caution.

Concept of Dual Methods

Implanon™ does not protect the user from sexually transmitted diseases (STDs). To decrease the risk of contracting or transmitting a STD, the user should insist that her male partner use a condom.

Discontinued Product

Norplant®

The Norplant® implant system was a progestin-based contraceptive medication formulated for 5 years of continuous use. The implant system consisted of six soft silastic implants each containing 36 mg of levonorgestrel (LNG) powder that was released to achieve a LNG level of 0.3 ng/mL. The implants were 34 mm long and 2.4 mm in diameter. They were placed in a fan-shaped arrangement into the subcutaneous tissue on the medial aspect of a woman's nondominant upper arm.

Although the Norplant® implant system was effective as a contraceptive, with a typical-use failure rate of 0.05%, the side effect of irregular vaginal bleeding led many to discontinue it. After placement of the implants, some bleeding was attributed to atrophy of the endometrium, but some was the result of ovulatory cycles. Because the circulating concentration of LNG was just above the level to inhibit ovulation, approximately one third of women were ovulating after 1 year of Norplant® use and two thirds were ovulating after 5 years of Norplant® use.

Improper placement made removal of Norplant® rods more difficult than anticipated. Some rods were placed too deep, and all six were not in the same plane, as would have facilitated their identification. Some women attributed somatic complaints of arm pain or sensory loss to a retained Norplant® implant. Because the Norplant® implant system was designed for a 5-year period of use, early discontinuation made Norplant® less cost effective.

In July 2002, Norplant®'s manufacturer, Wyeth Pharmaceuticals, announced that it would not resume sales of the implant system and renewed its offer to pay for removals through the end of the year.

References

1. Depo-Provera® contraceptive injection package insert. Pfizer Pharmaceuticals, Inc., New York, NY, 2004.

2. Breast cancer and depot-medroxyprogesterone acetate: a multi-national study. WHO Collaborative Study of Neoplasia and Steroid Contraceptives. *Lancet* 1991;338:833-838.

3. Jordan A: Toxicology of depot medroxyprogesterone acetate. *Contraception* 1994;49:189-201.

4. Berenson AB, Breitkopf CR, Grady JJ, et al: Effects of hormonal contraception on bone mineral density after 24 months of use. *Obstet Gynecol* 2004;103:899-906.

5. Cromer BA, Stager M, Bonny A, et al: Depot medroxyprogesterone acetate, oral contraceptives and bone mineral density in a cohort of adolescent girls. *J Adolesc Health* 2004;35: 434-441.

6. Lara-Torre E, Edwards CP, Perlman S, et al: Bone mineral density in adolescent females using depot medroxyprogesterone acetate. *J Pediatr Adolesc Gynecol* 2004;17:17-21.

7. Theintz G, Buchs B, Rizzoli R, et al: Longitudinal monitoring of bone mass accumulation in healthy adolescents: evidence for a marked reduction after 16 years of age at the levels of lumbar spine and femoral neck in female subjects. *J Clin Endocrinol Metab* 1992;75:1060-1065.

8. Naylor KE, Iqbal P, Fledelius C, et al: The effect of pregnancy on bone density and bone turnover. *J Bone Miner Res* 2000;15:129-137.

9. More C, Bettembuk P, Bhattoa HP, et al: The effects of pregnancy and lactation on bone mineral density. *Osteoporos Int* 2001; 12:732-737.

10. Sangi-Haghpeykar H, Poindexter III AN, Bateman L, et al: Experience of injectable contraceptive users in an urban setting. *Obstet Gynecol* 1996;88:227-233.

11. Matson SC, Henderson KA, McGrath GJ: Physical findings and symptoms of depot medroxyprogesterone acetate use in adolescent females. *J Pediatr Adolesc Gynecol* 1997;10:18-23.

12. Schwallie PC, Assenzo JR: Contraceptive use–efficacy utilizing medroxyprogesterone acetate administered as intramuscular injection once every 90 days. *Fertil Steril* 1973;24:331-339.

13. Amatayakul K, Sivasomboon B, Thanangkul O: A study of the mechanism of weight gain in medroxyprogesterone acetate users. *Contraception* 1980;22:605-622.

14. Martin HL Jr, Nyange PM, Richardson BA, et al: Hormonal contraception, sexually transmitted diseases, and the risk of heterosexual transmission of human immunodeficiency virus type 1. *J Infect Dis* 1998;178:1053-1059.

15. Gardner JM, Mishell DR Jr: Analysis of bleeding patterns and resumption of fertility following discontinuation of a long-acting injectable contraceptive. *Fertil Steril* 1970;21:286-291.

16. Garza-Flores J, Cardenas S, Rodriguez V, et al: Return to ovulation following the use of long-acting injectable contraceptives: a comparative study. *Contraception* 1985;31:361-366.

17. Implanon package insert. Organon USA, Inc. Roseland, NJ 2006.

Chapter 6

Intrauterine Contraception: Steroid- and Nonsteroid-based Devices

Although many different types of intrauterine devices (IUDs) are available worldwide, only two are available in the United States: the steroid-based Mirena®, which releases the progestin levonorgestrel (LNG), and the non-steroid-based ParaGard® T 380A, which releases copper. Use of IUDs has fallen in the United States because of product labeling changes, fear of litigation, and general misconceptions about IUD use. These factors, coupled with fewer health-care providers who have gained experience and confidence with IUD insertion, have contributed to fewer women using this contraceptive option.

Factors Influencing IUD Use

Product Labeling

Current prescribing information and package inserts for the two products available in the United States may influence providers and patients to restrict or avoid the use of an IUD for contraception. The prescribing information for the ParaGard® device recommends its use in women 'who have had at least one child, are in a stable, mutually monogamous relationship, and have no history of pelvic inflammatory disease (PID).'[1] The same wording is used in the Mirena® physician package insert, with the addition that the patient should 'have no history of ectopic pregnancy or condition that would predispose to ectopic pregnancy.'[2] These recommendations may be too restrictive. In a case-controlled study of 1,895 women, previous use of a copper IUD was not associated with an increased risk of tubal occlusion among nulligravid women (odds ratio [OR]=1, 95% confidence interval [CI] 0.5 to 1.6).[3] The presence of chlamydia antibodies and no IUD use was associated with infertility (OR=2.4, 95% CI 1.7 to 3.2). Although this study demonstrated no risk of tubal occlusion with copper IUD use, many health-care providers are reluctant to use a product outside recommended patient guidelines.

Fear of Litigation

In a national mailed survey of 811 practicing US obstetrician/gynecologists, 16% of respondents thought that performing IUD insertions put them at risk for litigation. Physicians who believed that IUD use led to litigation inserted significantly fewer IUDs in the preceding year than physicians who believed that IUDs did not lead to more litigation (4 vs 10, respectively, $P<0.001$).[4] In a review of claims against Planned Parenthood, only 18 (10%) involved IUDs, and only two resulted in unfavorable settlements. Both cases involved failure to diagnose PID and were unrelated to IUD use.[5]

6

Misconceptions About IUD Use

In the above survey, 20% of physicians thought that the IUD was an abortifacient, and 29% believed that IUDs increased the risk of PID by ≥10%.[4] Although its exact mechanisms of action are unclear, the IUD does not work as an obvious abortifacient. A primary mechanism seems to be the prevention of fertilization.[6] To verify the absence of occult conception cycles, Segal et al[7] examined serum human chorionic gonadotropin (hCG) levels in 30 IUD users for 30 months. He found no documented hCG production in these IUD subjects. This finding was confirmed with a highly sensitive urine assay in IUD users.[8] In a study by Alvarez et al,[9] washings from the uterus and fallopian tubes of women at the time of surgical sterilization at midcycle yielded fewer recovered oocytes from IUD users than from nonusers (39% vs 56%, respectively). Of the oocytes recovered from women who had intercourse before the sterilization procedure, normal cleaving embryos were found in women without IUDs but not in IUD users, suggesting a failure of sperm to fertilize the oocyte in IUD users.

Secondary mechanisms of action for the IUD involve its interactions with sperm, cervical mucus, and uterine contractions and the inhibition of implantation. The copper-containing IUD has been associated with altered normal uterine contractions that may lead to decreased sperm transport through the reproductive tract.[10] It seems to inhibit implantation by creating an inflammatory response with production of a cytotoxic endometrial cytokine.[11] The progestin-releasing IUD can thicken cervical mucus, leading to decreased sperm penetration and survival.[12] It also seems to inhibit implantation by creating an inflammatory response and by a direct progestin effect on the endometrium. The endometrial stroma becomes decidualized, glands become atrophic, and menstrual bleeding is decreased. In users of the progestin-releasing IUD, 75% of cycles are ovulatory, and bleeding patterns vary from amenorrhea to regular menstrual bleeding.[13] In a 3-year follow-up study of 165 women using Mirena®, 47% of patients were amenorrheic and the remainder had less dysmenorrhea.[14] In comparison, the copper-containing IUD is associated with a longer menses and a 50% increase in the amount of menstrual blood loss.[15]

With regard to increased risk for PID, there is only a transient increase in the incidence of infection for a short period after IUD insertion. A review of World Health Organization (WHO) clinical trial data found that immediately after IUD insertion, the incidence of PID was 9.7 cases/1,000 woman-years.[16] Twenty days after IUD insertion, the incidence dropped significantly to 1.6 cases/1,000 woman-years. The association between IUD insertion and infection is based on bacterial colonization of the uterus upon insertion. Use of a single dose of 200 mg doxycycline (Vibramycin®) or 500 mg azithromycin (Zithromax®) an hour before IUD insertion can decrease the incidence of PID. Similarly, the incidence of infertility is not linked to IUD use, but is more closely associated with the presence of antibodies to chlamydia.[3] Return to fertility after removal of an IUD is similar to that after discontinuation of other contraceptive methods (eg, oral contraceptive pills [OCPs], diaphragm).[17]

Steroid-based Intrauterine Device

Product Available in the United States

Mirena® Intrauterine System (Berlex Laboratories)
http://www.mirena-us.com
Toll-free telephone number: 1-888-Berlex-4 (1-888-237-5394)

6

The Mirena® device is a LNG-releasing IUD approved by the US Food and Drug Administration (FDA) in December 2000. Mirena® consists of a T-shaped polyethylene vertical stem with a reservoir containing 52 mg of LNG (Figure 6-1). Two monofilament threads are attached to a loop at the end of the vertical stem. Initially, LNG is released at a concentration of 20 μg/day. The amount decreases to 10 μg/day after the device's 5-year period of approved use. One small study, however, has suggested that Mirena® can remain in place for up to 7 years without loss of effectiveness.[18] The device contains barium sulfate, making it radiopaque.

Insertion

The Mirena® device is recommended to be inserted within 7 days of the onset of menstruation.[2] Many practitioners strictly adhere to this recommendation because the cervical canal is dilated at the time of menstruation, and the patient is less likely to have an occult pregnancy. Others have suggested that an IUD can be inserted at any time during the menstrual cycle, as long as the clinician is certain that the patient is not pregnant. If the Mirena® is

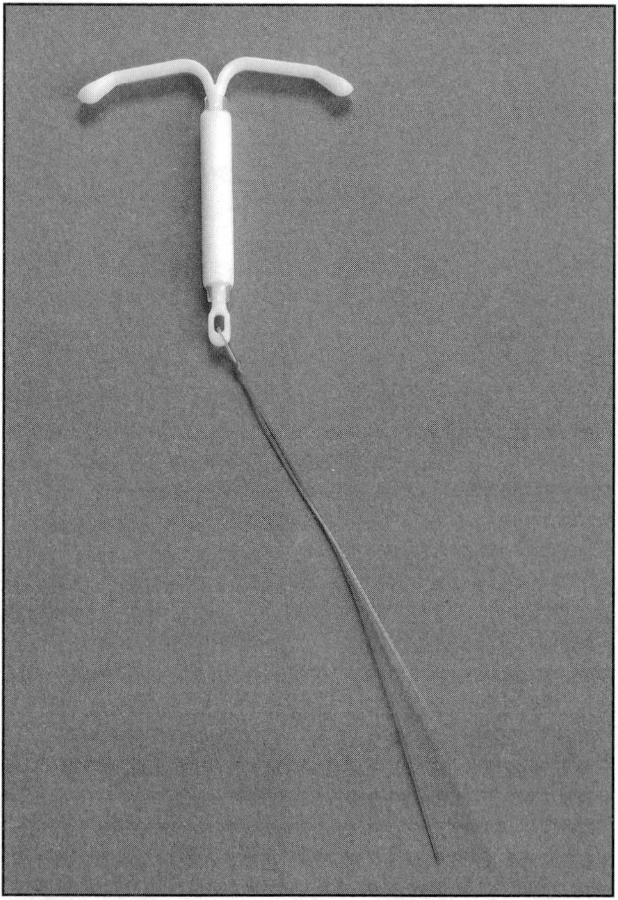

Figure 6-1: The Mirena® Intrauterine System (IUS).

inserted in the immediate postpartum period (<48 hours after delivery), there is an increased risk of expulsion. If it is placed in the postpartum period from 48 hours to <4 weeks, there is an increased risk of uterine perforation because the uterine walls are thinner in the typical early postpartum hypoestrogenic environment, and the progestin may slow uterine involution. After 4 weeks postpartum, Mirena® can be inserted with fewer of the above concerns. If a patient is breastfeeding, some progestin effect may be transferred to the infant until 6 weeks postpartum, and there is an increased risk for uterine perforation. Mirena® can be inserted after either a first- or second-trimester abortion, with some increased risk of expulsion and delayed uterine involution if placed after a second-trimester abortion.

Detailed instructions on placement of the Mirena® device can be found on the Mirena® Web site. A Mirena® insertion training video can also be obtained from a local company sales representative. To decrease uterine cramping during IUD insertion, ingestion of a nonsteroidal anti-inflammatory medication (eg, ibuprofen 400 to 800 mg) 30 to 60 minutes before insertion is often helpful. If cervical dilation is necessary to insert the IUD, a paracervical block can decrease the discomfort of the dilation procedure, or the patient can be given oral misoprostol (Cytotec®), and the IUD insertion performed in 12 hours. In a placebo-controlled study of nulliparous women, cervical dilation was greater and force to dilate the cervix was less 12 hours after administration of 400 μg misoprostol.[19]

Contraceptive Efficacy

The Mirena® device has a reported 5-year cumulative failure rate of 0.7 pregnancy/100 women.[2] When compared with all methods of female tubal sterilization procedures, which have a 5-year cumulative failure rate of 1.31 (95% CI 1.08 to 1.54) and a 10-year cumulative failure rate of 1.85/100 women (95% CI 1.51 to 2.18), the IUD is highly effective.[20] When a conception occurs, it is more likely to be an ectopic pregnancy because the IUD offers less protection against ectopic than intrauterine pregnancies. Because of an overall decline in pregnancies, the use of Mirena® does not increase the risk of ectopic pregnancy. The ectopic pregnancy rate is 0.22/100 women after 5 years of Mirena® use.[21]

Noncontraceptive Benefits

Progestin release often diminishes the patient's menstrual flow, and in a 3-year follow-up study of Mirena® users, 47% of patients were amenorrheic.[14] In a randomized, comparative study of Mirena® use vs endometrial resection for the symptom of menorrhagia, both treatments reduced menstrual bleeding after 1 year of treatment in a similar fashion.[22] Because hysteroscopic endometrial resection requires surgical expertise, a number of practitioners may find insertion of the Mirena® device easier to perform.

Side Effects

Some patients using the Mirena® device find the absence of menses worrisome and request removal of the device. Women should be counseled about the alterations in their menstrual cycles before insertion so they can prospectively consider this change.

A 5% chance of spontaneous IUD expulsion can be expected after insertion, with increased incidence expected when the placement is in the immediate postpartum period (<48 hours after delivery).[23] When the expulsion is undetected, it is often associated with contraceptive failure. Other risks include uterine perforation and failure to detect the IUD threads. Use of transvaginal ultrasound scanning and/or an abdominal radiograph has helped to verify the location of the IUD. If it has perforated the uterine wall, it should be removed and may require further surgical intervention.

Frequently Asked Questions

How can I insert an IUD in an obese patient when the direction of the uterine cavity is unclear?

To determine the direction of the uterine cavity in an obese patient, the concurrent use of transabdominal ultrasound scanning through a full bladder can help to facilitate the insertion of the IUD and verify its location.

Can you insert the Mirena® device in a patient with latex allergy?

The Mirena® device can be safely inserted into the uterus of a woman with a history of latex allergy.

Nonsteroid-based Intrauterine Device

Product Available in the United States

ParaGard® T 380A (FEI Women's Health LLC)
http://www.paragard.com
Automated response: 1-877-ParaGard
Toll-free clinician hotline: 1-800-319-0398

6

The ParaGard® T 380A is a T-shaped polyethylene IUD with a 68.7 mg copper sleeve on each of its transverse arms and 176 mg of copper wire wound around its vertical axis (Figure 6-2). The total surface area of copper is 380 mm^2. The tip of the vertical arm is enlarged to a 3-mm bulb, and two monofilament polyethylene threads are attached to the bulb. The IUD measures 36 mm along the vertical stem and 32 mm across the horizontal arms. It contains barium sulfate, which makes it radiopaque. The ParaGard® T 380A was approved by the FDA in 1984 and was introduced into clinical use in 1988. It is approved for 10 years of use, but it has been shown to be effective for 12 years.[24]

Insertion

The ParaGard® T 380A is recommended to be inserted in 'the latter part of the menstrual period, or 1 to 2 days thereafter.'[24] Similar to the Mirena® device, many practitioners insert the ParaGard® early in the menstrual cycle, when the cervical canal is dilated and the patient is less likely to have an occult pregnancy. The risks of postpartum device expulsion and uterine perforation are the same as for the Mirena®. Also, as with the Mirena®, the ParaGard® T 380A can be inserted after a first- or second-trimester abortion, with some increased risk of expulsion if placed after a second-trimester abortion.

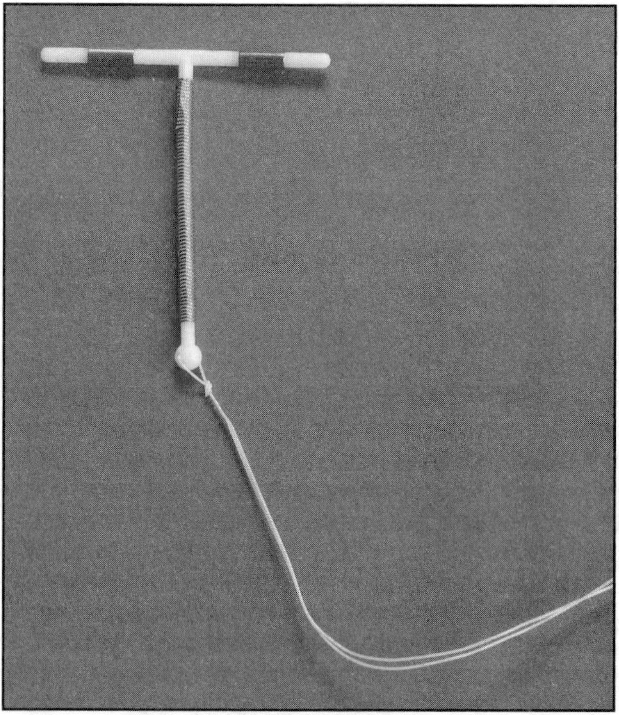

Figure 6-2: The ParaGard® T 380A.

Detailed instructions on placement of the ParaGard® can be found on the ParaGard® Web site. To decrease uterine cramping during IUD insertion, ingestion of a nonsteroidal anti-inflammatory medication before insertion is often helpful. If cervical dilation is necessary to insert the IUD, a paracervical block and/or taking oral misoprostol before insertion may be helpful.

Contraceptive Efficacy

The ParaGard® has a reported failure rate of 0.6 to 0.8 pregnancy/100 women.[1] Similar to the Mirena® device, when a conception occurs, it is more likely to be an ectopic pregnancy; however, use of ParaGard® does not increase the risk of ectopic pregnancy. The cumulative ectopic pregnancy rate is 0.89/100 women after 10 years of ParaGard® use.[25]

Noncontraceptive Benefits

Use of ParaGard® is associated with a decreased incidence of endometrial cancer.[26] The observed protective effect may be a result of copper's ability to initiate biochemical alterations that affect endometrial cellular response.

Side Effects

A major distinction between progestin- and copper-releasing IUDs is the effect on menstrual bleeding patterns. With a copper-releasing IUD, there is a prolongation of menses and a 50% increase in the amount of menstrual blood loss.[15] This bleeding pattern continues as long as the IUD is in place. After 1 year of use, serum ferritin levels are lower, suggesting depletion of iron stores and possible anemia.[27] This change is correctable with iron replacement therapy. The 5% incidence of spontaneous IUD expulsion, risk of possible uterine perforation upon IUD insertion, and failure to detect the IUD threads are similar to those of the Mirena® device.

Frequently Asked Questions

Can a patient with an allergy to copper use ParaGard® for contraception?

The package insert for the ParaGard® T 380A states that an allergy to copper is a contraindication to the use of this IUD for contraception.[1]

Must I remove my ParaGard® T 380A before an MRI examination?

The ParaGard® is not affected by magnetic resonance imaging (MRI).

References

1. ParaGard® T 380A intrauterine copper contraceptive prescribing information. FEI Women's Health LLC, North Todawanda, NY, 2003.

2. Mirena® package insert. Berlex Laboratories, Monteville, NJ, 2003.

3. Hubacher D, Lara-Ricalde R, Taylor DJ, et al: Use of copper intrauterine devices and the risk of tubal infertility among nulligravid women. *N Engl J Med* 2001;345:561-567.

4. Stanwood NL, Garrett JM, Konrad TR: Obstetrician-gynecologists and the intrauterine device: a survey of attitudes and practice. *Obstet Gynecol* 2002;99:275-280.

5. York SS: IUD litigation: the Planned Parenthood experience. *Am J Gynecol Health* 1989;3:35-37.

6. Rivera R, Yacobson I, Grimes D: The mechanism of action of hormonal contraceptives and intrauterine contraceptive devices. *Am J Obstet Gynecol* 1999;181:1263-1269.

7. Segal SJ, Alvarez-Sanchez F, Adejuwon CA, et al: Absence of chorionic gonadotropin in sera of women who use intrauterine contraceptive devices. *Fertil Steril* 1985;44:214-218.

8. Wilcox AJ, Weinberg CR, Armstrong EG, et al: Urinary human chorionic gonadotropin among intrauterine device users: Detection with a highly specific and sensitive assay. *Fertil Steril* 1987; 47:265-269.

9. Alvarez F, Brache V, Fernandez E, et al: New insights on the mode of action of intrauterine contraceptive devices in women. *Fertil Steril* 1988;49:768-773.

10. Maslow KD, Lyons EA: Effect of oral contraceptives and intrauterine devices on midcycle myometrial contractions. *Fertil Steril* 2003;80:1224-1227.

11. Ämmälä M, Nyman T, Strengell L, et al: Effect of intrauterine contraceptive devices on cytokine messenger ribonucleic acid expression in the human endometrium. *Fertil Steril* 1995;63: 773-778.

12. Jonsson B, Landgren BM, Eneroth P: Effects of various IUDs on the composition of cervical mucus. *Contraception* 1991;43:447-458.

13. Nilsson CG, Lahteenmaki P, Luukkainen T: Ovarian function in amenorrheic and menstruating users of a levonorgestrel-releasing intrauterine device. *Fertil Steril* 1984;41:52-55.

14. Baldaszti E, Wimmer-Puchinger B, Loschke K: Acceptability of the long-term contraceptive levonorgestrel-releasing intrauterine system (Mirena®): a 3-year follow-up study. *Contraception* 2003; 67:87-91.

15. Larsson G, Milsom I, Jonasson K, et al: The long-term effects of copper surface area on menstrual blood loss and iron status in women fitted with an IUD. *Contraception* 1993;48:471-480.

16. Farley TM, Rosenberg MJ, Rowe PJ, et al: Intrauterine devices and pelvic inflammatory disease: an international perspective. *Lancet* 1992;339:785.

17. Vessey MP, Lawless M, McPherson K, et al: Fertility after stopping use of the intrauterine contraceptive device. *Br Med J (Clin Res Ed)* 1983;4:179-184.

18. Sivin I, Stern J, Coutinho E, et al: Prolonged intrauterine contraception: a seven-year randomized study of the levonorgestrel 20 mcg/day (LNg 20) and the Copper T380 Ag IUDS. *Contraception* 1991;44:473-480.

19. Ngai SW, Chan YM, Liu KL, et al: Oral misoprostol for cervical priming in non-pregnant women. *Hum Reprod* 1997;12:2373-2375.

20. Peterson HB, Xia Z, Hughes JM, et al: The risk of pregnancy after tubal sterilization: findings from the US Collaborative Review of Sterilization. *Am J Obstet Gynecol* 1996;174:1161-1168.

21. Backman T, Rauramo I, Huhtala S, et al: Pregnancy during the use of levonorgestrel intrauterine system. *Am J Obstet Gynecol* 2004;190:50-54.

22. Istre O, Trolle B: Treatment of menorrhagia with the levonorgestrel intrauterine system versus endometrial resection. *Fertil Steril* 2001;76:304-309.

23. Grimes D, Schulz K, van Vliet H, et al: Immediate post-partum insertion of intrauterine devices: a Cochrane review. *Hum Reprod* 2002;17:549-554.

24. United Nations Development Programme: Long-term reversible contraception: twelve years of experience with the TCu380A and TCu220C. *Contraception* 1997;56:341-352.

25. Ganacharya S, Bhattoa HP, Batar I: Ectopic pregnancy among non-medicated and copper-containing intrauterine device users: a 10-year follow-up. *Eur J Obstet Gynecol Reprod Biol* 2003;111: 78-82.

26. Hubacher D, Grimes DA: Noncontraceptive benefits of intrauterine devices: a systematic review. *Obstet Gynecol Surv* 2002; 57:120-128.

27. Hassan EO, El-Husseini M, El-Nahal N: The effect of 1-year use of the CuT 380A and oral contraceptive pills on hemoglobin and ferritin levels. *Contraception* 1999;60:101-105.

Chapter 7

Emergency Contraception

Emergency contraception (EC) encompasses three different methods of contraception designed to prevent conception after unprotected sexual intercourse or after the failure of another contraceptive method. The original method, using combination oral contraceptive pills (OCPs), was described by Dr. Albert Yuzpe and was commonly referred to as the 'morning after pill.'[1] This method has been modified to use a progestin-only medication, but the concept of administering a high dose of steroids to decidualize the endometrium is essentially unchanged from its initial description. The US Food and Drug Administration (FDA) has approved one combination medication, the Preven® Emergency Contraceptive Kit (discontinued by the manufacturer in May 2004), and one progestin-only medication, Plan B®, for EC. A nonhormonal method of EC is to insert a copper-containing intrauterine device (IUD) to inhibit implantation. EC does not act as an abortifacient and will not disrupt an implanted pregnancy or act as a teratogen.

Information about EC can be found at:
http://www.not-2-late.com
Toll-free telephone number: 1-888-NOT-2-LATE (1-888-668-2528)

Combination Oral Contraceptive Pills

In the original Yuzpe method, two Ovral® (estrogen/progestin) combination OCPs were ingested within 72 hours of intercourse, and the dosage was repeated in 12 hours. The pregnancy rate for all regularly cycling patients exposed at midcycle was 1.4% (3/217). Some prominent side effects of this therapy were nausea and vomiting (51.7%) caused by the high estrogen content of the medication (50 μg of ethinyl estradiol [EE] per tablet; total estrogen amount per treatment, 200 μg of EE over 12 hours). To minimize nausea, it is recommended that patients use an antiemetic before ingesting Ovral®.[2]

Other combination OCPs have been used with similar effectiveness (Table 7-1). One uniquely packaged form of combination OCP was the Preven® Emergency Contraceptive Kit. This product contained four pills, two to be taken immediately and two to be taken 12 hours later. The manufacturer stopped production of Preven® in May 2004, but some residual kits may still be available at pharmacies. Preven® is still a safe and effective product. If available, it provides a convenient way of using a small number of combination OCPs to prevent pregnancy. In its place, other available combination OCPs can be used from an existing 28-day cycle pack. The advantage of using existing OCPs can be product availability or the patient's familiarity with taking OCPs. A different number of pills is given, depending on the strength of the progestin in each pill. The patient may need to ingest two to five pills per dose to consume a sufficient amount of progestin to decidualize the endometrium.

Progestin-only Method

To further decrease the side effects of nausea and vomiting, studies have investigated the ingestion of only a progestin for EC. In a randomized, controlled trial of the progestin levonorgestrel (LNG) vs a combination OCP, the LNG regimen was more effective and better tolerated than the combination OCP method.[3] The study was conducted in 1,955 women, and the crude pregnancy rate was 1.1% (11/976) in the LNG group vs 3.2% (31/979) in the combination OCP group. The crude relative risk (RR) of pregnancy between the two methods was 0.36 (95%

Table 7-1: Combination Oral Contraceptive Pills (OCPs) Used for Emergency Contraception (EC)

Trade Name	Number and Color of Pills Taken Initially	Number and Color of Pills Taken After 12 Hours
Alesse®	5 pink	5 pink
Levlen®	4 light orange	4 light orange
Levlite®	5 pink	5 pink
Levora®	4 white	4 white
Lo/Ovral®	4 white	4 white
Low-Ogestrel®	4 white	4 white
Nordette®	4 light orange	4 light orange
Ogestrel®	2 white	2 white
Tri-Levlen®	4 yellow	4 yellow
Triphasil®	4 yellow	4 yellow
Trivora®	4 pink	4 pink

Modified from American College of Obstetricians and Gynecologists (ACOG). Emergency oral contraception, *ACOG Practice Bulletin* 25, Washington, DC, ACOG, 2001.

7

confidence interval [CI] 0.18 to 0.70). An estimated 85% of pregnancies were prevented using the LNG method vs 57% using the combination OCP method. The side effects of nausea (23.1% vs 50.5%) and vomiting (5.6% vs 18.8%) were both significantly reduced (P <0.01) in the LNG group compared with the combination OCP group. The decrease in these two side effects was attributed to the absence of estrogen in the LNG method.

Similarly, progestin-only pills (Ovrette®) containing the progestin norgestrel (NRG) have been used for EC. Because the dose of progestin contained in these pills is low (0.075 mg NRG/pill), the protocol calls for 20 pills to be ingested immediately and the dose repeated in 12 hours. The use of desogestrel (DSG) and norgestimate (NGM), progestins used in combination OCPs, as single agents for EC has not been studied.

FDA-approved Protocol

Plan B® (Duramed Pharmaceuticals, Inc.)
http://www.go2planb.com
Toll-free telephone number: 1-800-330-1271

The availability and simple packaging of Plan B® have made this product much easier to use than other progestin-only methods. In a recent study, investigators examined whether the two 0.75 mg doses of LNG used in Plan B® could be combined in a single 1.5 mg dose without loss of efficacy. The study was a randomized, double-blind trial in 15 family planning clinics in 10 countries. Each arm of the study had 1,356 subjects included in the efficacy analysis. The pregnancy rates were 1.5% and 1.8% in the women assigned one- and two-dose LNG, respectively. There were no significant differences in pregnancy rates and side effects between the two methods.[4] In another study, it was estimated that using just one Plan B® tablet (0.75 mg LNG) within 1 hour of inadequately protected sexual intercourse would be associated with a failure rate of only one pregnancy in 700 exposures (failure rate of 0.14%).[5]

On August 24, 2006, the FDA approved the sale of Plan B® to women ≥18 years without a prescription. Women <17 years would be able to obtain Plan B®, but only by prescription. To monitor proper distribution, Plan B® can only be dispensed to licensed drug wholesalers, pharmacies, or clinics with licensed health-care practitioners. The product cannot be displayed and must be kept behind the pharmacy counter. After patient request and age verification, the product can be dispensed.

Insertion of a Copper-containing IUD

The insertion of a copper-containing IUD, ParaGard® T 380A, preferably within 5 days of inadequately protected intercourse, can prevent pregnancy and be used for ongoing contraception. Upon insertion, the copper-containing IUD disrupts implantation by creating an inflammatory response with the production of a cytotoxic endometrial cytokine.[6] The IUD can be inserted up to 8 days after intercourse if ovulation is known to occur 3 or more days after coitus. The failure rate of this method is estimated to be <0.1%.[7] Selection of patients for insertion of the ParaGard® T 380A should follow the selection guidelines discussed in Chapter 6. In general, this method should be reserved for women who wish to continue using the IUD as their primary mode of contraception.

Other Protocols

Another EC option may be the off-label use of the antiprogestin mifepristone, also known as RU-486 or Mifeprex®, which is approved for the termination of early pregnancy. Additional background information on this medication is discussed in Chapter 13. Mifepristone is not approved for EC, but limited studies have demonstrated effectiveness. In a study of 800 women requesting EC, 398 received the standard combination OCP therapy of two doses of 100 μg of EE and 1 mg of NRG, 12 hours apart.[8] The remaining 402 women received 600 mg of mifepristone. Medications were given within 72 hours (3 days) of exposure to sperm. No conceptions occurred in the mifepristone group, and four conceptions occurred in the OCP group, which was not statistically significant. There was less nausea (40% vs 60%) and vomiting (3% vs 17%) with mifepristone compared with standard OCP EC, but there was a delay in the onset of next menstrual period with mifepristone. In a multicenter, single-masked, dose-response study, 1,717 women were randomized to receive 600, 50, or 10 mg of mifepristone.[9] This trial was conducted in 11 family planning clinics in Australia, China, Finland, the Republic of Georgia, the United Kingdom, and the United States. A similar number of pregnancies (7, 6, and 7) occurred with the three doses (600, 50, and 10 mg, respectively). The authors suggested that 10 mg of mifepristone might be just as effective for EC as the higher doses. In comparison, when 10 mg of mifepristone was used for contraception either weekly or within 5 days of exposure to sperm, the conception rate was unacceptably high and the study was terminated prematurely (see Chapter 13). When evaluating research trials of medication for EC, study findings may be biased if the exposure to sperm is not uniform and the chance of conceiving is dissimilar among study participants.

Frequently Asked Questions

What can I use for nausea when I'm taking two birth control pills?

To prevent nausea associated with EC, patients can use nonprescription drugs such as meclizine hydrochloride (Bonine®, Dramamine® II), taking one or two 25 mg tablets 1 hour before the first EC dose and repeating, if needed, in 24 hours. Patients can also use cyclizine lactate taking one 50 mg tablet 30 minutes before the first EC dose and repeating as needed every 4 to 6 hours, or the antihistamine diphenhydramine hydrochloride (Benadryl®), taking one to two 25 mg tablets or capsules 1 hour before the first EC dose and repeating as needed every 4 to 6 hours.

If I vomit after taking the medication, should I take another dose?

The patient should take another dose of EC only if she vomits within 1 hour of the dose or she can see the pills in the emesis.

References

1. Yuzpe AA, Smith RP, Rademaker AW: A multicenter clinical investigation employing ethinyl estradiol combined with dl norgestrel as postcoital contraceptive agent. *Fertil Steril* 1982;37:508.

2. Raymond EG, Creinin MD, Barnhart KT, et al: Meclizine for prevention of nausea associated with use of emergency contraceptive pills: a randomized trial. *Obstet Gynecol* 2000;95:271-277.

3. Randomised controlled trial of levonorgestrel versus the Yuzpe regimen of combined oral contraceptives for emergency contraception. *Lancet* 1998;352:428-433.

4. Von Hertzen H, Piaggio G, Ding J, et al: Low dose mifepristone and two regimens of levonorgestrel for emergency contraception: a WHO multicentre randomised trial. *Lancet* 2002;360:1803-1810.

5. Shelton JD: Repeat emergency contraception: facing our fears. *Contraception* 2002;66:15-17.

6. Ämmälä M, Nyman T, Strengell L, et al: Effect of intrauterine contraceptive devices on cytokine messenger ribonucleic acid expression in the human endometrium. *Fertil Steril* 1995;63:773-778.

7. Trussell J, Ellertson C: Efficacy of emergency contraception. *Fertility Control Reviews* 1995;4:8-11.

8. Glasier A, Thong KJ, Dewar M, et al: Mifepristone (RU 486) compared with high-dose estrogen and progestogen for emergency postcoital contraception. *N Engl J Med* 1992;327:1041-1044.

9. Task Force on Postovulatory Methods of Fertility Regulation: Comparison of three single doses of mifepristone as emergency contraception: a randomised trial. *Lancet* 1999;353:697-702.

Chapter 8

Barrier Contraception: Male Condoms

Condoms are barriers worn over the penis to prevent semen and sexually transmitted diseases (STDs) from coming into contact with a partner's orifice (eg, vagina, anus, mouth). Condoms have been shown to decrease the transmission rate of human immunodeficiency virus (HIV) 10-fold.[1,2]

Types and Sizes of Condoms

Condoms are usually made of latex, but can also be derived from polyurethane or natural animal membranes (eg, lamb cecum). Natural animal membranes may not provide the same degree of protection from STDs as condoms derived from synthetic materials. Polyurethane is a thin, soft, pliable plastic. Polyurethane condoms are more likely to slip and break than latex condoms because they do not adhere to the penis as well as latex does. Condoms can vary in thickness from 0.03 to 0.09 mm.

Condoms are available in various sizes, lengths, and widths at www.condomania.com (800-9-CONDOM, 800-926-6366). Other manufacturers offer condoms with different textures, spermicidal coating, lubricant, colors, flavors, and scents at www.ansellcondoms.com and www.askdurex.com.

Contraceptive Efficacy

In typical use, a condom's failure rate is estimated to be 15% (see Appendix A). Although the theoretic failure rate is much lower (2%), the higher typical-use failure rate is attributed to failure to use a condom with every ejaculation.[3] Condoms with a spermicidal coating have not been found to be more effective, and they are more expensive, with a shorter period of usefulness compared with nonmedicated condoms because of the expiration of the spermicide.

Proper Use of a Male Condom

A condom should be used with every coital event in the vagina, anus, or mouth. Latex condoms should be stored in a cool, dry place away from sunlight because latex can deteriorate with heat and humidity. The condom should be used as follows:

1. Check the expiration date on the package and do not use after that date. If only a production date is listed, condoms with a spermicide can be used for 2 years, and nonmedicated condoms for 5 years.
2. Open the condom package carefully, attempting to avoid ripping the condom. Squeezing the condom out of the package is often helpful.
3. Pull back the foreskin of the penis if the user is not circumcised.
4. Position the condom on the penis so the condom rolls downward.
5. Leave a half-inch space of condom to collect the semen. Pinch the air out of the end of the condom. Smooth out any air bubbles that may appear between the condom and the penis.
6. If desired, a user can apply a water- or silicone-based lubricant to a latex condom.
7. After ejaculation, withdraw the penis before the erection is lost. Hold the base of the condom with one hand against the shaft when withdrawing the penis to prevent loss of semen.
8. Inspect the condom for breaks.
9. Dispose of the condom, and never reuse a condom for intercourse.

10. Wipe any remaining ejaculate from the penis. Wash the penis with soap and water.
11. Use a new condom if the penis is inserted into a different orifice (vagina, anus, or mouth).

Step-by-step video instructions on proper condom use are available on Planned Parenthood's Web site www.ppfa.org under the heading 'health info.'

Concept of Dual Methods

To help prevent STDs, the female partner should insist that her male partner use a condom even if she is using a steroid-based or other method of contraception. This additional contraceptive precaution is termed the use of dual methods. Although this concept sounds good in theory, many young women who are at greatest risk do not follow it. In one study of women 15 to 24 years, only 7% used condoms with another contraceptive method.[4] If a male using a latex condom desires to have vaginal intercourse with a woman wearing a female polyurethane (plastic) condom, each condom may be less effective. Because of friction created between the two methods, either condom could break or slip despite the liberal use of lubricant.

Side Effects

When using a latex condom, either partner may have an allergic or hypersensitive response to the latex powder and/or the spermicide used with the condom. This reaction may escalate with an increased number of exposures to the latex. Using a plain polyurethane condom can avoid a patient's sensitivity to latex. A woman could also use the polyurethane female condom (see Chapter 9).

If a condom breaks or slips off during ejaculation in the vagina, emergency contraception (EC) could be started if the patient is at risk of conceiving. Immediate use of Plan B® (levonorgestrel [LNG]) and insertion of a spermicide into the vagina can help to prevent conception.

Cost of the Contraceptive Product

Condoms may be obtained free of charge or at a reduced rate at some public health centers. The average unit price for a latex condom is 50 cents. Polyurethane condoms range in price from 80 cents to $2.00. The price per condom decreases significantly to 4 to 6 cents when purchased in bulk directly from the manufacturer.

Frequently Asked Questions

What lubricants can and cannot be used with latex condoms?

With latex condoms, safe, appropriate lubricants include water, saliva, K-Y Jelly, Astroglide®, Gynol II®, or silicone lubricant. Inappropriate (oil-based) lubricants that interact with the latex condom and lead to breaks include baby oil, vegetable oil, suntan lotion, and mineral oil. If a patient still wants to use one of these inappropriate lubricants, then the male partner should use a polyurethane condom that can resist them.

How do some condoms delay ejaculation?

Some condom manufacturers have added benzocaine to their lubricated condoms. It desensitizes the nerve endings in the penis to help delay penile ejaculation. This addition has helped men with a history of premature ejaculation delay emission. One manufacturer, Durex, places the benzocaine cream inside the tip of the condom, and it disperses with body heat. The company sells this condom under the brand-name Performax.

What can be done to correct a loss of penile sensation when using a condom?

To increase penile sensation, a thinner or larger condom may help. Often, the condom may be too small, too thick, or incompletely unrolled. Applying more lubricant to the outside of the condom will help to increase sensation and reduce friction when penetrating the orifice. This will also help to maintain a penile erection.

References

1. Pinkerton SD, Abramson PR: Effectiveness of condoms in preventing HIV transmission. *Soc Sci Med* 1997;44:1303-1312.

2. Davis KR, Weller SC: The effectiveness of condoms in reducing heterosexual transmission of HIV. *Fam Plann Perspect* 1999;31: 272-279.

3. Steiner MJ, Cates W Jr, Warner L: The real problem with male condoms is nonuse. *Sex Transm Dis* 1999;26:459-462.

4. Raine T, Minnis AM, Padian NS: Determinants of contraceptive method among young women at risk for unintended pregnancy and sexually transmitted infections. *Contraception* 2003;68:19-25.

Chapter 9

Barrier Contraception: Diaphragm, Cervical Cap, and the Female Condom

The Diaphragm

The diaphragm is a latex rubber device designed to fit over the cervix and keep spermicide in close contact with cervical mucus. Its mechanism of action is to function as a barrier to sperm, and the spermicide acts as a vaginal microbicide to kill sperm. The diaphragm is dome shaped to contain the spermicide, and some modifications have been made to help it maintain its position between the symphysis pubis and the posterior fornix.

Before insertion, the distance between the symphysis pubis and the posterior fornix should be estimated to choose the correct-sized diaphragm. Diaphragms are available only by prescription from a health-care provider. Because the diaphragm is composed of latex rubber, oil-based or greasy substances may cause deterioration. The substances to avoid include cocoa butter, cold cream, petroleum jelly, mineral oil, and vegetable oil.

Concept of Dual Methods

Use of a diaphragm does not protect the user from sexually transmitted diseases (STDs). To decrease the risk of contracting or transmitting a STD, the user should insist that her male partner use a condom.

Side Effects

Use of a diaphragm may be associated with an increased incidence of urinary tract infections (UTIs), especially if the diaphragm is not fitted properly. Women with symptoms of a UTI should be examined and have the size of their diaphragm confirmed by a health-care provider.

Products Available in the United States

Ortho All-Flex® Arcing Spring Diaphragm (Ortho-McNeil Pharmaceutical, Inc) http://www.orthowomenshealth.com

The Ortho All-Flex® Arcing Spring diaphragm is made of a natural rubber. It has a dual spring-within-a-spring construction that allows the diaphragm to arc no matter where the rim is compressed. This feature allows for better occlusion of the cervix in women with pelvic relaxation (eg, mild cystocele, rectocele) or retroversion of the uterus. The diaphragm is available in diameters from 55 to 95 mm in 5-mm increments. It was introduced in the United States in 1940.

Contraceptive Efficacy

In a 6-month study examining the contraceptive efficacy of the Ortho All-Flex® diaphragm using 2% nonoxynol-9 (N-9) spermicide, the typical-use pregnancy probability was 7.9%.[1] It is generally accepted that the 1-year typical-use pregnancy rate using a diaphragm is approximately 16% to 20% (see Appendix A).[2]

Proper Use

The Ortho All-Flex® diaphragm should be inserted as follows:

1. Have the patient squat or stand with a foot up on a chair. Insert a finger into the vagina to locate the cervix. Instruct users that the cervix is soft and has the consistency of a person's nose.
2. Fill the diaphragm with 2 tsp of spermicide (approximately two-thirds full).
3. Squeeze the Ortho All-Flex® diaphragm together between the finger and thumb. Insert the diaphragm

with bowl facing upward and push it upward toward the cervix. Position the Ortho All-Flex® diaphragm to cover the cervix.

4. After ejaculation, the diaphragm must stay covering the cervix for at least 6 hours and not longer than 24 hours.

The Ortho All-Flex® diaphragm should be removed as follows:

1. Have the user squat or perform Valsalva's maneuver to help bring the diaphragm down into the vagina.
2. Insert one finger into the bowl of the diaphragm to draw it down the vagina for removal.
3. Wash the diaphragm with a mild liquid soap and water and then pat it dry. The diaphragm should be replaced every 2 years or sooner if it shows signs of wear or deterioration. To prolong the life of a diaphragm, a user can lightly dust it with cornstarch.

A user of the Ortho All-Flex® diaphragm should have the diaphragm size checked if she has had a weight change of 10 pounds, used the diaphragm for 1 year, given birth, or had an abortion.

Frequently Asked Question

Since I don't use my diaphragm often, do I have to replace it in a year?

Because the Ortho All-Flex® Arcing Spring diaphragm is made of rubber, it has a limited lifespan regardless of use. It should be replaced every 2 years, or sooner if it has been exposed to excessive sunlight or temperatures. If the rubber diaphragm deteriorates quickly under normal use, consider using a silicone diaphragm (Wide-Seal® silicone diaphragm), which is more durable.

Ortho® Coil Spring Diaphragm
(Ortho-McNeil Pharmaceutical, Inc.)
http://www.orthowomenshealth.com

The Ortho® Coil Spring diaphragm is made of natural rubber. It is held in place by a tension-adjusted, cadmium-plated coil spring. The spring allows the diaphragm to be

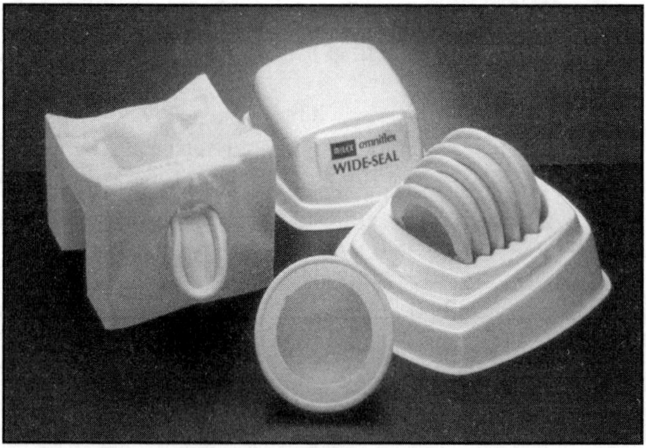

Figure 9-1: The Wide-Seal® silicone diaphragm.

compressed into one plane and inserted with the Ortho Universal Diaphragm Introducer or with the user's fingers. The diaphragm is available in diameters from 55 to 95 mm in 5-mm increments. Introducers can only be used with diaphragm sizes between 60 and 90 mm. The Ortho® Coil Spring diaphragm was introduced in the United States in 1940. The instructions for use and associated efficacy are similar to those for the Ortho All-Flex® diaphragm.

Wide-Seal® Silicone Diaphragm
(Milex Products, Inc.)
http://www.milexproducts.com
Toll-free telephone number: 1-800-621-1278

The Wide-Seal® diaphragm from Milex Products, Inc. has a wider rim that provides more surface contact with the vagina to prevent the diaphragm from dislodging during intercourse (Figure 9-1). Because the diaphragm is made of silicone, it is hypoallergenic, does not absorb odors or secretions, and lasts longer than rubber diaphragms. The Wide-Seal® diaphragm comes in two versions, the arcing and the omniflex diaphragms, which are similar to the Ortho All-Flex® and the Ortho® Coil Spring diaphragm, respectively. The Wide-Seal® diaphragms are not available at pharmacies and must be purchased directly from the company. The instructions for use of the Wide-Seal® diaphragm and its associated efficacy are similar to those of the Ortho All-Flex® diaphragm.

The Cervical Cap

Similar to the diaphragm, cervical cap barrier methods coupled with the use of a spermicide require a woman to be highly motivated if she is using the device as her primary method of contraception. Because of the cervical cap's smaller size and lesser compression of the bladder, there may be a lesser incidence of UTIs than with the diaphragm. Because the efficacy of the cervical cap depends on its covering of the cervix, any cervical cap in the immediate postpartum and postabortal period may be less effective because of the enlargement of the cervix during these periods. Studies have demonstrated that the cervical cap is less effective in parous vs nulliparous women.[1,3] As with other barrier methods, users should be informed of the availability of emergency contraceptive (EC) methods should their barrier method fail or they choose not to use it.

Concept of Dual Methods

The cervical cap does not protect against STDs. To decrease the risk of contracting or transmitting a STD, the user should insist that her male partner use a condom.

Products Available in the United States

FemCap™ (FemCap, Inc.)
http://www.FemCap.com
Toll-free telephone number: 877-4-FemCap (877-433-6227)

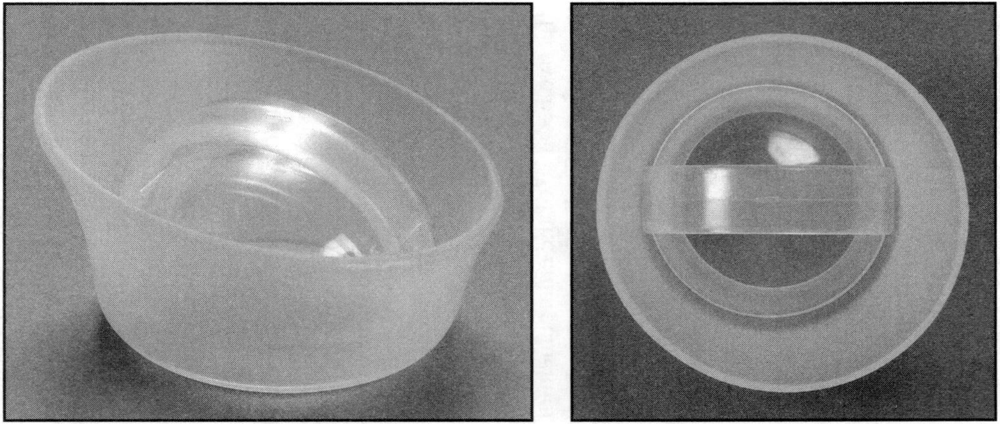

Figure 9-2: The FemCap™ cervical cap.

FemCap™ is a silicone (latex-free) reusable cervical cap approved for use in April 2003 by the US Food and Drug Administration (FDA) (Figure 9-2). It is available in three sizes (determined by the inner diameter of the rim): 22 mm for nulligravid women, 26 mm for women who have been pregnant but not had a vaginal delivery, and 30 mm for women who have had a vaginal delivery of a full-term baby.

Contraceptive Efficacy

In a 6-month study comparing the FemCap™ cervical cap with the Ortho All-Flex® diaphragm, both using N-9 spermicide, the typical-use pregnancy probabilities were 13.5% and 7.9%, respectively.[1] There was a trend for a greater chance of conception if the user had a previous delivery (15.8%) than if she had no previous deliveries (9.5%). In the FemCap™ package insert, the 1-year pregnancy probabilities were projected from the above 6-month barrier study. The 1-year chance of pregnancy using all sizes of the FemCap™ was estimated to be 23%.[4] When the three sizes of the FemCap™ were considered individually, the 22-mm, 26-mm, and 30-mm cervical caps were associated with an estimated 14%, 14%, and 29% 1-year chance of pregnancy, respectively.

Proper Use

The FemCap™ should be inserted as follows:

1. Have the patient squat and insert a finger into the vagina to locate the cervix.
2. Place approximately 1/4 tsp of spermicide in the bowl of the FemCap™ (the side that will face the cervix).
3. While holding the removal strap, spread a thin layer of spermicide over the outer rim.
4. Place approximately 1/2 tsp of spermicide in the groove between the rim and the dome of the FemCap™ (side with removal strap will face into the vagina).
5. Squeeze the FemCap™ with finger and thumb. Insert squeezed cap with bowl facing upward and the long rim entering first.

6. Push the FemCap™ down toward the rectum and back toward the cervix. Position the FemCap™ over the cervix so the long rim points toward the rectum, and press inward to seal it against the cervix.
7. After ejaculation, the FemCap™ must stay covering the cervix for at least 6 hours and not longer than 48 hours.
8. If vaginal intercourse is planned within the 6-hour period, check the position of the FemCap™ by finger palpation before intercourse. Do not remove the FemCap™, just insert the spermicide into the vagina. Insert another 1/2 tsp of spermicide before ejaculation.
9. The FemCap™ should be removed after 48 hours to prevent an increased risk of toxic shock syndrome.

The FemCap™ should be removed as follows:

1. To facilitate removal, have the patient squat and perform Valsalva's maneuver to bring the cervix closer to the introitus.
2. Push the dome of the FemCap™ with a finger to break the suction and allow grasping of the removal strap.
3. With gentle traction, pull the FemCap™ out of the vagina.
4. Wash the FemCap™ with antibacterial hand soap and water. Rinse it with water and pat it dry. Store the FemCap™ in its provided storage container.

Step-by-step instructions and an animated video on insertion and removal of the FemCap™ are also available on the manufacturer's Web site. In addition, a videotape of the insertion technique and a package insert accompany each FemCap™ cervical cap. The FemCap™ should be replaced after 2 years, or sooner if deterioration occurs.

Side Effects

Use of the FemCap™ may increase the frequency of vaginal infections and UTIs.

Frequently Asked Question

Since FemCap™ is made of silicone instead of latex rubber, can I use my FemCap™ when I'm treating myself for a yeast infection?

Although the FemCap™ is made of silicone that would resist deterioration from petroleum-based medications, it should not be used during a vaginal infection. Another form of contraception that does not reside in the vagina should be used (eg, male condom), and the woman should see her health-care provider to treat the vaginal infection.

Lea's Shield® Vaginal Barrier Contraceptive Device (Yama Inc.)
http://www.leasshield.com
E-mail: info@leasshield.com
Toll-free telephone number: 1-800-699-8130

Lea's Shield® is a silicone rubber reusable cervical cap available in only one size with a valve to vent the cap and facilitate its placement (Figure 9-3). It was approved by the FDA in March 2002. The cap is shaped like an elliptical bowl (55 mm at its widest point, total weight=38 g) with an anterior loop to help in removal. The thicker posterior end fits into the posterior vaginal fornix and stabilizes the cup by inhibiting its rotation. Located on the top of the cup is a one-way valve that allows air to escape during placement, thus creating a suction effect against the cervix. Uterine and cervical fluids can be released into the vaginal canal, but sperm cannot enter. Despite its one-way valve, Lea's Shield® should not be used during a woman's menses. Lea's Shield® should not be used when vaginal or cervical lacerations or vaginal, cervical, and pelvic infections exist. The manufacturer states that Lea's Shield® differs from other cervical caps in that it is held in place by the vaginal walls covering the cervix and not by the cervix itself. The one-way valve helps to facilitate a close approximation over the cervix.

Contraceptive Efficacy

In a study of 146 women using Lea's Shield® with and without 3% N-9 spermicide in a double-blind fashion, the 6-month life-table pregnancy rates were 5.6% and 9.3%, respectively (P=0.086), when controlled for age, center, and frequent prior use of barrier methods.[1] There was a

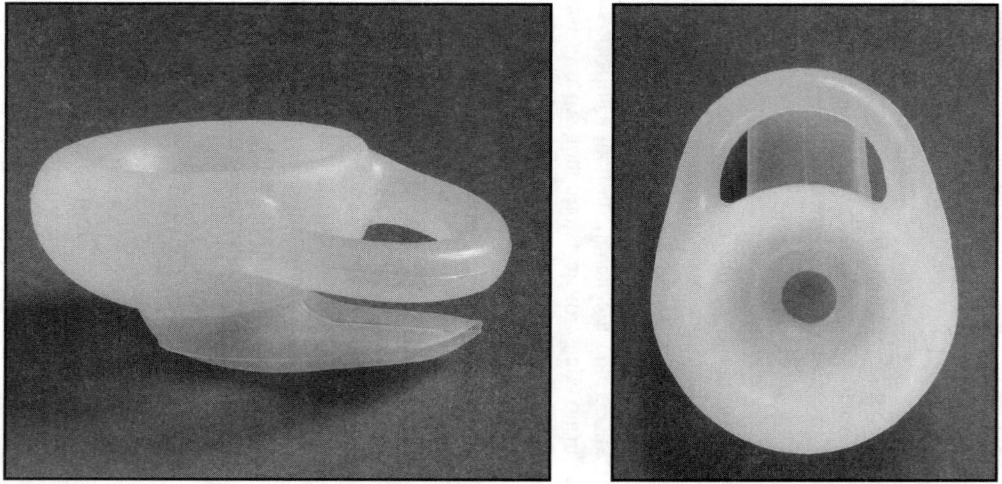

Side

Top

Figure 9-3: The Lea's Shield® cervical cap.

higher failure rate in parous than in nulliparous women. In this study, 84% of the patients were parous, and parity alone may have contributed to a higher than expected failure rate. Although this study was performed with and without spermicide, Lea's Shield® should be used with nonoxynol-9 spermicide.

In a study of 59 women who used Lea's Shield® with 3% N-9 for 6 months as their only form of birth control, the pregnancy rate was 8.79%. Based on the 6-month trial data, the projected failure rate after 1 year was 15%.[5]

Proper Use

Lea's Shield® should be inserted as follows:

1. Have the patient squat and insert a finger into her vagina to locate the cervix. Instruct her that the cervix is soft and has the consistency of a person's nose.
2. Coat the inside of the Lea's Shield® bowl with spermicide. Do not overfill the bowl. Place a small amount of spermicide along the leading edge of the bowl to facilitate insertion of Lea's Shield®. Also coat the outer part of the valve. Use a total of about 2 tsp of spermicide.
3. Squeeze the Lea's Shield® together between the finger and thumb. Insert the squeezed cap with the bowl facing upward and the thicker portion (opposite side of loop) entering first.
4. Push the Lea's Shield® upward in the vagina toward the cervix. Position it covering the cervix, and press inward to seal it against the cervix.
5. After ejaculation, Lea's Shield® must stay covering the cervix for 8 hours and not longer than 48 hours.

Lea's Shield® should be removed as follows:

1. Have the user squat or perform Valsalva's maneuver to help bring the Lea's Shield® down in the vagina.
2. Grasp the loop of the Lea's Shield® with the fingers and twist until the suction is broken (sounds like a pop). The patient can also insert one finger into the bowl to break the suction and remove the cervical cap.

Table 9-1: Adverse Effects Reported With Use of Lea's Shield®

Effect	Percentage
Male partner pain or discomfort caused by the device	8.2%
Female partner pain or discomfort caused by the device	6.6%
Abnormal bleeding or spotting	6%
Vaginitis	4.4%
Abnormal Pap test	3.9%
Urinary tract infection (UTI)	3.8%

3. Pull down on loop of Lea's Shield® to remove it from the vagina.
4. Wash the Lea's Shield® with a mild liquid soap and water for approximately 2 minutes and then pat it dry. It should be stored in its silk pouch. Lea's Shield® should be replaced if it shows signs of wear or deterioration.

Side Effects

In a study of 182 users, 34.6% (63 of 182) reported serious and/or unexpected adverse events that were possibly or probably related to the use of Lea's Shield®.[4] The most common events are listed in Table 9-1. Because the device is used with a spermicide, there are also reports of the spermicide causing vaginal irritation.

Frequently Asked Question

Lea's Shield® appears to work like a diaphragm, but diaphragms come in different sizes. Why does Lea's Shield® come in only one size?

Lea's Shield® and the diaphragm do work similarly to occlude the cervical opening and hold spermicide in close approximation to the cervix, but they differ in how they are positioned in the vagina. Lea's Shield® is held against the cervix by the vaginal walls, and the one-way valve helps to vent any air or secretions to create a close approximation to the cervix. The bowl of Lea's Shield® is wide enough to accommodate the dimensions of most women's cervices. The diaphragm is held between the symphysis pubis and the posterior fornix, a dimension that varies among women. To size the diaphragm properly, this distance should be measured by an experienced examiner and requires a pelvic examination.

Prentif™ Cavity-Rim Cervical Cap (Cervical Cap Ltd.)
http://www.naturalgynae.com
Telephone number: 408-395-2100

The Prentif™ Cavity-Rim Cervical Cap is a latex rubber, reusable, cervical cap available in four sizes: 22 mm, 25 mm, 28 mm, and 31 mm, as measured across the internal rim diameter (Figure 9-4). Along the inner surface of the Prentif™ rim, there is a narrow groove that can create a seal when the cap is placed over the cervix, thus providing a physical barrier against oocyte fertilization. The cap is used in conjunction with spermicide that is placed inside it. The Prentif™ cervical cap is approximately 1.5 inches long and is held in place by suction and the support of the vaginal walls. The Prentif™ cervical cap was approved by the FDA in May 1988. It is manufactured in England and distributed exclusively in the United States by Cervical Cap Ltd.

If a male latex condom is used, the condom may become attached or 'grab onto' the Prentif™ cervical cap. Using a lubricant to coat the outside of the condom may prevent this problem.

The Prentif™ Cavity-Rim Cervical Cap can be obtained from a health-care provider or the US distributor. If the health-care provider does not have the cervical cap in stock, it can be obtained from the distributor, but it must be shipped to the prescribing health-care provider or a pharmacy. Detailed ordering instructions are available on the company's Web site, as is a ZIP code listing of providers.

Proper Use

The Prentif™ cervical cap must be prescribed and fitted by a health-care provider. It should not be used in a woman with an unusually shaped cervix caused by prior cervical lacerations, surgery, scarring, or any variation that leads to a less-optimal occlusion of the cervix by the cap. It should not be used in women with unresolved abnormal Pap smears, or current vaginal or cervical infections. If a patient is having her menstrual period or unscheduled uterine bleeding, she should not use the Prentif™ cervical cap. Because the Prentif™ cervical cap is made of latex rubber, vaginal medications that contain petroleum may cause it to deteriorate. The Prentif™ cervical cap should not be used until the vaginal treatment is completed.

When choosing the proper size of the Prentif™ cervical cap, examine the woman during her periovulatory period (midcycle) when the cervix is slightly smaller. This will ensure an optimal fit at the most important time during the menstrual cycle. In the period after a term delivery, women should wait 6 weeks before using a cervical cap. Women who have had a first trimester elective or spontaneous abortion should be fitted for the Prentif™ cervical cap 2 weeks after the abortion.

The Prentif™ cervical cap should be inserted as follows:

1. Have the patient squat or stand with a foot up on a chair. Insert a finger into the vagina to locate the cervix.
2. Fill the Prentif™ cervical cap one third full with spermicide. Do not coat the rim of the Prentif™ cervical cap.
3. Separate the labia with one hand and with the other squeeze the rim of the cap between the thumb and index finger.

4. Slide the cap up the vagina and position it over the cervix.
5. Press the rim of the cap around the cervix until it is completely covered. Confirm placement by sweeping a finger around the rim of the cap. No cervix should be felt outside the cap. The dome of the cap should indent, but not collapse. After a minute, test the suction of the cap on the cervix by attempting to pull the dome off the cervix. The cap should not separate from the cervix with gentle traction.
6. After ejaculation, the Prentif™ cervical cap must stay covering the cervix for at least 8 hours and not longer than 48 hours.
7. Insertion of additional spermicide with repeated acts of intercourse within a 40-hour period while the cap is in place is not required.

The Prentif™ cervical cap should be removed as follows:

1. Have the user squat and perform Valsalva's maneuver or stand with one foot up on a chair to facilitate locating the cap covering the cervix.
2. Insert two fingers into the vagina and press on the rim of the cap until the suction is broken. Grasp the cap and remove it from the vagina.
3. Wash the cap with a mild liquid soap and water. Air or pat the cervical cap dry. To prolong the life of a Prentif™ cervical cap, lightly dust it with cornstarch.

After 3 months of Prentif™ cervical cap use, the physician should do the following:

1. A pelvic examination with a Pap smear to detect any abnormal change in the Pap smear. Before the Pap smear, the patient should not use her cervical cap for 2 to 3 days.

After 12 months of Prentif™ cervical cap use, the following should be done:

1. Perform a pelvic examination with a Pap smear. The FDA and the manufacturer recommend that the Prentif™ cervical cap be replaced yearly.

Contraceptive Efficacy

According to the package insert, the Prentif™ Cavity-Rim Cervical Cap has a range of effectiveness from 82.6% to 93.6%. The effectiveness varies 'depending on consistency of use.' No other specific information concerning efficacy studies is readily available.[6]

Frequently Asked Questions

When I remove the Prentif™ cervical cap, I notice dark blood inside the cap. What should I do?

Blood within the cap may be caused by menstrual bleeding or unscheduled uterine bleeding, or be a sign that the cap is not fitting properly or is becoming dislodged during intercourse. The cervix can bleed if the cap does not cover it completely and causes contact bleeding at the edge of the cervix. The Prentif™ cervical cap should not be used during menses or when uterine bleeding is present because of the possible increased incidence of toxic shock syndrome.

What lubricants must I avoid if I use the Prentif™ cervical cap?

Because the Prentif™ cervical cap is composed of latex rubber, oil-based or greasy substances may cause deterioration of the rubber. The substances to avoid include cocoa butter, cold cream, petroleum jelly, mineral oil, or vegetable oil.

How can I stop my Prentif™ cervical cap from having a foul odor?

A foul odor may be a sign of a vaginal infection. Users with this sign should see their health-care provider for an examination. If no infection exists, wearing the cap for a shorter time or using a different spermicide may decrease the odor. Users who add a spermicide cream rather than a gel notice a rancid odor accompanying their cap with prolonged use. Soaking the cap in a bactericidal mouthwash (eg, Listerine®) may also be helpful.

I've noted some vaginal irritation when I'm using the Prentif™ cervical cap. What could this be from?

Vaginal irritation could be a sign of a vaginal infection, and a pelvic examination is warranted. If no infection is

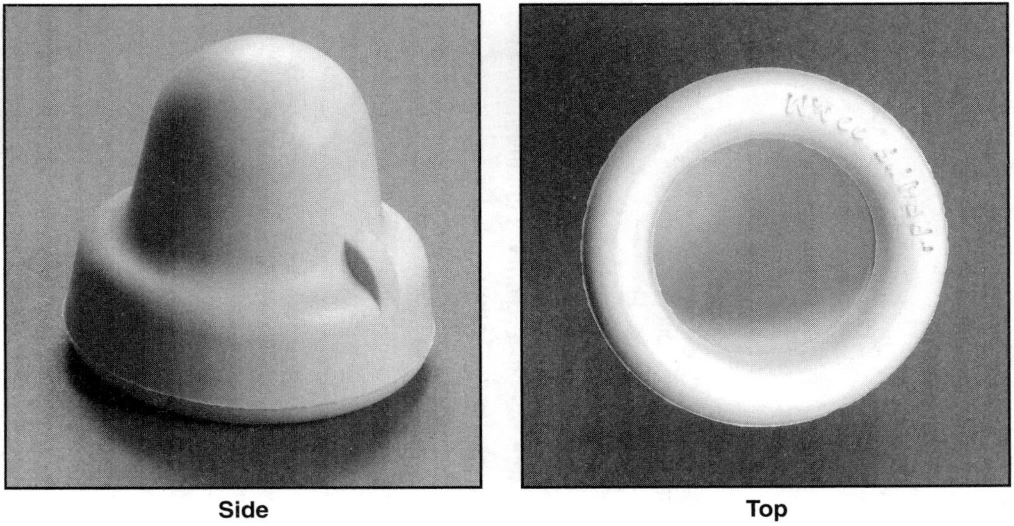

Figure 9-4: The Prentif™ Cavity-Rim Cervical Cap.

found, the irritation may be from the spermicide. Vaginal irritation is more pronounced in women using the stronger 3% N-9 contraceptive jelly preparation (eg, Ortho Options® Gynol II® Extra Strength) rather than the 2% formulations. The irritation may also be more prominent when using it in a cervical cap for 48 hours than when inserting it into the vagina.

The Female Condom

To give women more choices of barrier contraceptives and additional protection against the spread of STDs, the concept of a protective sheath encompassing the entire vagina and a portion of the perineum has been developed. Women can insert the female condom up to 8 hours before intercourse.

Products Available in the United States

FC Female Condom®, Reality® Female Condom (The Female Health Company) http://www.femalehealth.com, Toll-free telephone number: 1-800-635-0844

The FC Female Condom® is a female-initiated barrier method of contraception and disease prevention. It is made of polyurethane and is suitable for couples when the male has a latex allergy and does not want to use a polyurethane male condom. The condom is 17 cm long (approximately 6.5 inches) and has a flexible ring at each end of the sheath. The inner ring at the closed end is inserted into the vagina, similar to a diaphragm, and the outer ring is placed over the perineum. The condom is prelubricated with a silicone-based, nonspermicidal lubricant to facilitate insertion. In the United States, the FC Female Condom® is sold under the brand-name Reality® Female Condom. It is approved by the FDA for 5 years from the manufacture date.

Contraceptive Efficacy

In a large study in the United States and Latin America to assess the efficacy and acceptability of the FC Female

Condom®, the 6-month pregnancy rate was 2.6% in the United States sites and 9.5% in the Latin American sites.[7] In a similar study in Japan with 190 women, the 6-month life-table probability of conceiving was 3.2% during typical use and 0.8% during correct and consistent use of the product.[8]

Noncontraceptive Benefits

In addition to its contraceptive efficacy, the female condom can prevent STDs in a fashion similar to the male condom.[9]

Proper Use

The condom should be used in the following manner:

1. Open the package by tearing at the notch in the upper right-hand corner. Use of a scissors to cut open the package may damage the condom.
2. Insert the condom while squatting, sitting at the edge of a chair, raising one foot on the seat of a chair, or lying on one's back.
3. Hold the sheath at the closed end and squeeze the flexible inner ring (like a diaphragm) between the thumb and second or middle finger. The condom is now squeezed together for easier insertion.
4. Insert the inner ring into the vagina, and position the ring behind the pubic bone.
5. Using the middle finger, insert it into the inside of the condom and place the inner ring up into the vagina as far as possible. Do not twist the sheath of the condom. The outer ring should rest on the outside of the vagina partially covering the perineum.
6. Guide the head of the penis into the sheath. The shaft of the penis should be covered by the condom sheath on all sides.
7. The patient may use an additional water-, silicone-, or oil-based lubricant to decrease friction during intercourse. Use of a lubricant can decrease the noise created by the female condom moving in the vagina.

8. After ejaculation, twist the outer ring of the condom to seal it and to help retain any secretions within the condom. With some gentle traction, the condom is easily pulled out of the vagina.
9. Inspect the condom for breaks.
10. Wrap the condom in its package or toilet tissue and discard in the trash. Do not flush it down the toilet.

Step-by-step instructions on proper female condom use are also available on the manufacturer's Web site www.femalehealth.com. Patients should practice inserting the female condom before use because one study suggested that 25% of women were unable to insert the product after practicing the insertion on a plastic model.[10]

An off-label use of this product would be to clean and reuse it for another coital event to prevent conception. Reuse of this product may not protect the user from STDs as well as a single use does. The manufacturer has applied for official approval to reuse the female condom. Steps to reuse the female condom outlined by the World Health Organization (WHO) are as follows:

1. Make a weak bleach solution of 1 part bleach to 20 parts of water. This will kill viruses and bacteria such as human immunodeficiency virus (HIV) and gonococcus.
2. Soak the female condom in the weak bleach solution for 1 minute.
3. Rinse the condom with water.
4. Wash with soap and water and pat dry.
5. Store at room temperature in a dry place.
6. May reuse up to five times. More information can be obtained from the WHO Information Update at the Web site www.who.int/reproductive-health/stis/docs/report_reuse.pdf.

Concept of Dual Methods

When a woman chooses to use the female condom, in addition to the contraceptive benefit, she is also protecting herself from STDs. The additional STD protection fulfills the concept of practicing dual methods.

Side Effects

Use of the female condom may increase the frequency of vaginal infections and UTIs.

Frequently Asked Question

The female condom appears to be too large for the vagina. How will it fit?

The female condom appears to be large, but it is similar in length to an unrolled male condom, with the exception that it is wider. The wider outer opening may be less restrictive than a male condom, which is a complaint of some male condom users. When the inner ring of the female condom is pinched together and the condom gathered together for insertion, the female condom fits easily inside the vagina, leaving the outer ring to partially cover the perineum.

The Contraceptive Sponge

Overview

The Today's® Sponge is a polyurethane, single-size, over-the-counter contraceptive product that contains the spermicide N-9 (1 g/sponge). It was introduced in the United States in 1983 and was withdrawn in 1995 because of manufacturing deficiencies. Rather than upgrade its production plant, the manufacturer, American Home Products, decided to suspend sales of the contraceptive. The FDA has never questioned the safety or efficacy of the Today's® Sponge. In 1998, Allendale Pharmaceuticals acquired the patents and the manufacturing equipment to produce the Today's® Sponge. In April 2005, it obtained FDA approval for marketing in the United States.

The Today's® Sponge is moistened with approximately 2 tbs of water and squeezed once. It is placed high in the vagina covering the cervix. The sponge should be positioned with the dimple side toward the cervix and the woven polyester removal loop facing outward. It must be inserted 30 minutes before intercourse and left in place for a minimum of 6 hours and a maximum of 30 hours. One sponge is protective against repeated coital episodes during a 24-hour period. Prolonged sponge use is associated with vaginal infections and possible toxic shock syndrome. The sponge has perfect- and typical-use failure rates of 9% and 16%, respectively, in nulliparous women (see Appendix A). In parous women, the failure rates are increased to 20% and 32%, respectively. The higher failure rate in parous women has been attributed to the increased size of the parous vs the nulliparous cervix. Similar to a diaphragm, the sponge does not protect the user from STDs. To decrease the risk of contracting or transmitting a STD, the user should insist that her partner use a condom.

References

1. Mauck C, Callahan M, Weiner DH, et al: A comparative study of the safety and efficacy of FemCap™, new vaginal barrier contraceptive, and the Ortho All-Flex® Diaphragm. *Contraception* 1999;60:71-80.

2. Ortho All-Flex® Diaphragm (Web page). Ortho-McNeil Pharmaceutical, Inc. Web site. Available at: http://www.orthowomenshealth.com.

3. Mauck C, Glover LH, Miller E, et al: Lea's Shield: a study of the safety and efficacy of a new vaginal barrier contraceptive used with and without spermicide. *Contraception* 1996;53:329-335.

4. FemCap™ package insert. FemCap, Inc., Del Mar, CA, 2003.

5. Lea's Shield® package insert. Yama, Inc., Millburn, NJ, 2002.

6. Prentif ™ Cavity-Rim Cervical Cap package insert. Cervical Cap Ltd., Los Gatos, CA, 2002.

7. Trussell J, Sturgen K, Strickler J, et al: Comparative contraceptive efficacy of the female condom and other barrier methods. *Fam Plann Perspect* 1994;26:66-72.

8. Trussell J: Contraceptive efficacy of the Reality® female condom. *Contraception* 1998;58:147-148.

9. French P, Latka M, Gollub E, et al: Use-effectiveness of the female versus male condom in preventing sexually transmitted diseases in women. *Sex Transm Dis* 2003;30:433-439.

10. Artz L, Demand M, Pulley L, et al: Predictors of difficulty inserting the female condom. *Contraception* 2002;65:151-157.

Chapter 10

Other Contraceptive Methods

Abstinence

Abstinence, or the prevention of any genital contact that may result in a pregnancy, is one form of contraception practiced by some individuals. The advantage of this method is that it is a self-motivated lifestyle change that can be initiated or reinitiated at any time. If the woman is in a relationship, she must have an understanding male partner who shares her desire to be abstinent. The disadvantage of this method is its drop in efficacy when practiced intermittently without a backup method of contraception. If women want to use this technique, they should be informed of the availability of emergency contraception (EC) and have condoms (male or female) available if they want to have sexual intercourse.

The term abstinence may have different meanings to different individuals. For some, abstinence is not having any type of sexual experience. For others, it may be more loosely defined and mean not having oral, anal, or vaginal intercourse. Others exclude any penetration of the vagina and anus, but believe oral/genital contact is acceptable.

In lieu of vaginal intercourse, some couples practice outercourse, in which they express their affection by kissing, hugging, massaging, mutual masturbation, and breast and nipple stimulation. With outercourse, there is no penetration of the vagina or anus, and no semen, vaginal fluids, or blood products are shared between the partners.

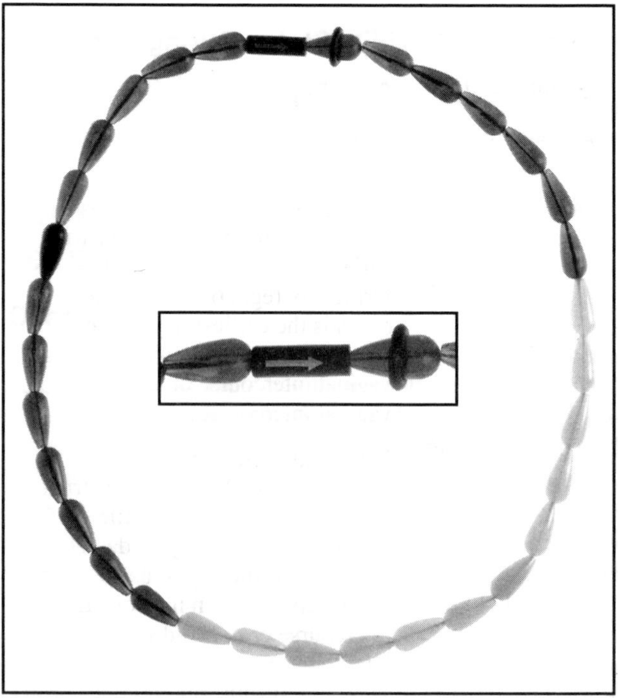

Figure 10-1: CycleBeads™.

Standard Days Method™

CycleBeads™ (Cycle Technologies)

http://www.cyclebeads.com

The concept of the calendar method is the basis for the Standard Days Method™ (SDM). This method uses CycleBeads™, which are a set of color-coded beads that display and track the fertile period of cycle days 8 through 19 (Figure 10-1). Because the beads representing the fertile period are predetermined, only women who have regular menstrual cycles every 26 to 32 days should use this method.

The Institute for Reproductive Health provided the financial support for the concept of the SDM with CycleBeads™. The Institute for Reproductive Health is located within the Department of Obstetrics and Gynecology at Georgetown University in Washington, DC. Further information about the Institute can be obtained from its Web site www.irh.org, by telephone (1-202-687-1392), or by e-mail (rhinfo@georgetown.edu).

Contraceptive Efficacy

In a prospective, multicenter trial in a heterogeneous population (N=478) aged 18 to 39 years, the cumulative probability of pregnancy was 4.75% and 11.96% over 13 cycles of perfect use and typical use, respectively.[1] This research was conducted in Bolivia, Peru, and the Philippines. Before the introduction of this method, the Institute for Reproductive Health familiarized 5 to 10 health workers (service providers) at each site with the SDM and the research study protocol. Women and, when possible, their partners were educated about the SDM and the use of the CycleBeads™. Participants in the research study were an average age of 29.4 years, were educated (85.1% had some secondary education or higher, 91% literate), and had at least one child (98.9%), and 55.9% had used the calendar method of natural family planning before. During the study, there were 43 pregnancies; 42% occurred during the first three cycles of CycleBeads™ use for contraceptive planning.

Proper Use

The CycleBeads™ are a connected string of 32 beads in which each bead represents a day of the menstrual cycle (Table 10-2). To assist women in determining their fertile period, the CycleBeads™ are used in the following manner:

1. On cycle day 1, the first day of menstrual bleeding, a movable, tight-fitting rubber ring is positioned on the red bead.
2. The rubber ring is moved one bead/day until it is positioned on a white bead, consistent with the beginning of the fertile period.

Table 10-2: Understanding CycleBeads™

Bead Number	Bead Color
1	Red
2-7	Brown
8-19	White
20-26	Brown
27	Dark brown
28-31	Brown
32	Brown

3. During the fertile period, cycle days 8 through 19, women should avoid having unprotected vaginal intercourse.
4. On cycle day 20, the rubber ring is positioned on a brown bead, signaling the less fertile period and a low probability of conceiving.
5. If the user starts her menstrual flow before cycle day 27 (eg, a cycle <26 days), or if her menses does not start by cycle day 32, she should contact her health-care provider for further instructions. If menses has not started by cycle day 32, the possibility of a recent conception should be excluded by a pregnancy test.

In the research study by Arévalo et al,[1] women who had two cycles outside the 26- to 32-day frequency were advised to use another contraceptive method and were withdrawn from the study. Women who did not have menses by cycle day 32 were tested for pregnancy.

Significance to Menstrual Cycle	Fertility Status
Cycle day 1, first day of menses	Not fertile
Cycle days 2-7	Not fertile
Cycle days 8-19	Fertile period
Cycle days 20-26	Not fertile
Cycle day 27; contact health-care provider if menses begins before this day	Not fertile
Cycle day 28-31	Not fertile
Cycle day 32; contact health-care provider if menses has not started by this day	Possible pregnancy

Withdrawal Method

10

In the withdrawal method, the male partner withdraws his penis completely outside the vagina before ejaculation. This method is also referred to as coitus interruptus. This method requires that the male partner sense when he is beginning to climax before his ejaculation.

Contraceptive Efficacy

In couples who use the withdrawal technique, the lowest expected failure rate is 4%, and the typical-use failure rate is 27% (see Appendix A). In some selected populations, the withdrawal method is more effective. Vessay et al[2] reported only a 7% failure rate, based on 674 woman-years of withdrawal use and 45 unintended pregnancies. Although the withdrawal method can be less effective than some barrier contraceptive techniques, it is better than no method at all and unprotected ejaculation in the vagina.

Couples using the withdrawal method should be advised of the availability of EC.

Failures with the withdrawal technique are attributed to the escape of preejaculatory fluid containing sperm into the vagina and cervical mucus. Sperm is not evenly distributed in a man's semen emission, with higher concentrations found in the first portion of the ejaculate. Two small studies have questioned the presence of large amounts of sperm in the pre-ejaculate. One study found no sperm in the pre-ejaculatory fluid of 16 men.[3] The other study found only a few clumps of sperm in 33% (5/15) of the men examined. The sperm isolated from these individuals appeared inactive.[4] If the withdrawal method is used properly, the number of failures seems to be minimized.

Proper Use

The withdrawal method is as follows:

1. Wipe off preejaculatory penile discharge before inserting the penis into the vagina.
2. Use a coital position that will allow the male partner to withdraw easily.

Couples could practice the withdrawal method with a barrier contraceptive in place to help the male partner learn self-control measures to prevent ejaculation, and to improve communication between partners. If a couple has intercourse soon after a first ejaculation, sperm may still be present in the penis and any preejaculate fluid. The withdrawal method may be less effective when the male partner has consumed alcohol that may impair his control of his ejaculation.

Concept of Dual Methods

The withdrawal method does not protect the user from STDs. To decrease the risk of contracting or transmitting a STD, the male partner should use a condom. The withdrawal method is best suited to couples in a mutually monogamous relationship.

Spermicides

Nonoxynol-9 Spermicide

Almost all available spermicides contain nonoxynol-9 (N-9), which achieves its contraceptive action from the ability to damage the sperm cell membrane. If the spermicide fails, the pregnancy is unaffected by it. Spermicide can be used alone, but is more effective when used with a condom or diaphragm. N-9 spermicides are available in a number of formulations—foam, cream, gel, suppositories, and film.

Contraceptive Efficacy

The contraceptive efficacy of the different spermicides available depends more on the amount of N-9 per dose than on the formulation of the N-9. In a prospective randomized study comparing three different doses of N-9 in a gel preparation with a film and a suppository, the lowest dose N-9 gel (52.5 mg) was less effective than the other gels (100 and 150 mg of N-9), film (100 mg of N-9), or suppository (100 mg of N-9).[5] In this study, the probability of pregnancy through 6 months of typical use was 22% in the 52.5 mg gel group, 16% in the 100 mg gel group, 14% in 150 mg gel group, 12% in the 100 mg film group, and 10% in the 100 mg suppository group.

A higher general failure rate was observed in a second prospective, randomized, multinational study comparing a 72 mg N-9 spermicidal film with a 100 mg N-9 foaming tablet.[6] The 6-month probability of pregnancy during typical spermicide use was 25% for the film group and 28% for the foaming-tablet group. The estimated 12-month cumulative probability of pregnancy was 39.8% in the film group and 44% in the foaming-tablet group. Although these rates are higher than those previously reported for spermicide use, this study was performed in countries where the fertility rates are higher than in the United States. The participants were 18 to 35 years, more likely to be married, had at least one child, and reported about 13 coital acts per 30-day interval. Prior studies have suggested that the 1-year failure rate associated with spermicide use is approximately 18% in perfect use and 29% in typical use (see Appendix A).

Products Available in the United States

The products listed below are representative of the types of available spermicides and do not constitute a complete list.

Ortho Options® Delfen® Vaginal Contraceptive Foam (Ortho-McNeil Pharmaceutical, Inc.)

Delfen® vaginal contraceptive foam is a greaseless, nonstaining, white contraceptive product sold in an aerosol container. The foam is transferred to an applicator and inserted into the vagina 1 hour before sexual intercourse. Each filled applicator contains 85 mg of N-9 12.5%.

Proper Use

Delfen® foam should be used in the following manner:

1. Shake can before each use.
2. Place can upright on a level surface and attach the applicator to the top of the can.
3. Press the applicator down to fill it with foam to the bottom of the ribbed section.
4. Remove applicator and insert into the vagina to dispense the foam around the cervix.
5. If coitus occurs again within 1 hour of prior foam application, add one more applicator of foam.
6. If coitus is planned for later than 1 hour after the first foam application, another applicator of foam must be inserted before sexual intercourse.

Ortho Options® Conceptrol® Gel (Ortho-McNeil Pharmaceutical, Inc.)

Conceptrol® gel is a clear, unscented, unflavored, stainless gel that contains 100 mg of N-9 4%. The gel is packaged in prefilled, single-dose, disposable plastic applicators.

Proper Use

The gel is used in the following manner:

1. Remove applicator from packaging, and insert into the vagina to dispense the gel around the cervix.
2. If coitus occurs again within 1 hour of prior gel application, add one more applicator of gel.
3. If coitus is planned for later than 6 hours after the first gel application, another applicator of gel must be inserted before sexual intercourse.

Ortho Options® Gynol II® Contraceptive Jelly (Ortho-McNeil Pharmaceutical, Inc.)

Gynol II® contains 100 mg of N-9 2% per applicator and is usually used with a diaphragm. The jelly is clear, unscented, water soluble, greaseless, and nonstaining. An additional applicator of contraceptive jelly should be inserted into the vagina if a second coital act occurs or if vaginal intercourse occurs more than 6 hours after insertion of the jelly. This product also comes in an extra-strength formulation (150 mg of N-9 3% per applicator).

Advantage-S® Bioadhesive Gel (Columbia Laboratories, Inc.)

Advantage-S® bioadhesive gel contains 52.5 mg of N-9 in an unscented, unflavored, nonstaining, polycarbophil-based, bioadhesive vaginal gel. This gel is reported to have increased adherence to the cervix, allowing a reduction in the amount of N-9 required for contraception in an effort to decrease vaginal epithelial irritation. The product is available in a prefilled, single-use applicator or in a tube with a reusable applicator.

In a randomized study, the 52.5 mg gel was less effective than two other gels that contained 100 and 150 mg of N-9 (see Contraceptive Efficacy above).[5]

Proper Use

Advantage-S® bioadhesive gel in a disposable applicator should be used in the following manner:

1. Grip applicator at thick end and shake downward (like a thermometer) to move contents to the thin end.
2. Twist off tab at thin end, and insert into vagina as deep as comfortably possible.
3. Press the thick end to squeeze the gel into the vagina.
4. Advantage-S® can be inserted 1 hour before intercourse.
5. An additional applicator of Advantage-S® is required for each act of vaginal intercourse.
6. Douching and bathing are not recommended immediately after using Advantage-S®. If the user wants to douche or bathe, she should wait at least 6 hours after the last intercourse for full spermicidal activity.

Encare® Vaginal Contraceptive Inserts (Thompson Medical Co. Inc.)

Encare® vaginal contraceptive inserts contain 100 mg of N-9/insert. Some users state that the suppositories do not melt entirely or disperse evenly.

Proper Use

Encare® oval suppositories should be used in the following manner:

1. Unwrap the suppository.
2. Insert the suppository into the vagina, using the fingers, and push it to the top of the vagina near the cervix.
3. Contraceptive protection begins 10 to 15 minutes after the insertion of the suppository and lasts no longer than 1 hour.

Ortho Options® Conceptrol® Foaming Tablets (Ortho-McNeil Pharmaceutical, Inc.)

Conceptrol® foaming tablets contain 100 mg of N-9/tablet. Users of the tablets sometimes find that the tablets become messy, and there are complaints of increased vaginal wetness. Some women do not like the effervescence of the foaming tablets.

Proper Use

Conceptrol® foaming tablets should be used in the following manner:

1. Insert the tablet, and push it to the top of the vagina.
2. To ensure that the tablet dissolves, it should be inserted 10 to 15 minutes before vaginal intercourse.

VCF® Vaginal Contraceptive Film™ (Apothecus, Inc.)
http://www.apothecus.com
Toll-free telephone number: 1-800-227-2393

VCF® Vaginal Contraceptive Film™ contains 72 mg of N-9/film. The film is 2 inches square and is slightly thicker than plastic wrap. Users find the film to be a more discreet and cleaner alternative to foam.

Proper Use

VCF® Vaginal Contraceptive Film™ should be used in the following manner:

1. Remove the film from its pouch and fold it in half.
2. Insert the film with a dry finger, and place the film at the top of the vagina near the cervix. Fingers should be dry to decrease the likelihood of the film adhering to the fingers.
3. VCF® should be inserted at least 15 minutes and not more than 3 hours before vaginal intercourse. A minimum of 15 minutes is required to ensure that the film has dissolved.
4. VCF® lasts approximately 3 hours, and a new film should be inserted before every ejaculation of semen into the vagina.

Concept of Dual Methods

Spermicide products do not protect the user from STDs. To decrease the risk of contracting or transmitting a STD, the user should insist that her male partner use a condom.

Side Effects

N-9 users may complain of a vaginal burning sensation or irritation. During oral/genital contact, some couples complain of an unpleasant taste or tingling of the oral mucous membranes.

N-9 spermicide is an epithelial irritant that may increase the disruption of the vaginal epithelium and possible ulceration. This epithelial irritation increases directly with frequent use of N-9. Evidence suggests that if the vaginal epithelium is weakened, N-9 may increase the acquisition of human immunodeficiency virus (HIV) and other STDs. In one study of Nairobi prostitutes, Kreiss et al[7] linked use of contraceptive sponges containing N-9 to increased genital ulcers and vulvitis that may have led to an increased transmission of HIV. However, this study may have had methodologic deficiencies leading to biases that overestimated the risk of HIV infection among N-9 users.

Studies are now ongoing to identify new spermicides that protect against conception and STDs without associated vaginal and/or cervical irritation.

Frequently Asked Question About Spermicides

What alternatives are there to N-9 spermicide?

There are two alternatives to N-9 spermicide—octoxynol-9 and benzalkonium chloride. Octoxynol-9 is available in the United States, as Koromex® cream and Ortho Options® Ortho-Gynol® jelly (not Gynol II® contraceptive jelly). In Canada, benzalkonium chloride is available as Pharmatex® spermicide.

References

1. Arévalo M, Jennings V, Sinai I, et al: Efficacy of a new method of family planning: the Standard Days Method. *Contraception* 2002;65:333-338.

2. Vessay M, Lawless M, Yeates D: Efficacy of different contraceptive methods. *Lancet* 1982;1:841-842.

3. Ilaria G, Jacobs JL, Polsky B, et al: Detection of HIV-1 DNA sequences in pre-ejaculatory fluid. *Lancet* 1992;340:1469.

4. Pudney J, Oneta M, Mayer K, et al: Pre-ejaculatory fluid as potential vector for sexual transmission of HIV-1. *Lancet* 1992;340: 1470.

5. Raymond EG, Chen PL, Luoto J, et al: Contraceptive effectiveness and safety of five nonoxynol-9 spermicides: a randomized trial. *Obstet Gynecol* 2004;103:430-439.

6. Raymond E, Dominik R: Contraceptive effectiveness of two spermicides: a randomized trial. *Obstet Gynecol* 1999;93:896-903.

7. Kreiss J, Ngugi E, Holmes K, et al: Efficacy of nonoxynol-9 contraceptive sponge use in preventing heterosexual acquisition of HIV in Nairobi prostitutes. *JAMA* 1992;268:477-482.

Chapter 11

Female Sterilization

Female sterilization is an important contraceptive option for many couples. In a 1998 report of trends in contraceptive use from 1982 to 1995, 27% of reproductive-aged women had undergone tubal occlusion procedures.[1]

Many methods exist to occlude the fallopian tubes. Although female sterilization is effective, the ultimate success of the sterilization depends on the type of procedure performed, the duration of surveillance after sterilization, and the age of the patient when sterilized. In a multicenter, prospective cohort study, 10,685 women who underwent tubal sterilization in US teaching centers were followed for 8 to 14 years.[2] There were 143 sterilization failures during the observation period. The 5- and 10-year probabilities of pregnancy were, for all methods, 13.1 pregnancies/1,000 procedures (95% confidence interval [CI] 10.8 to 15.4) and 18.5/1,000 procedures (95% CI 15.1 to 21.8), respectively (Table 11-1). The tubal occlusions were grouped into six general classes: bipolar coagulation, unipolar coagulation, silicone rubber band application, spring clip application, interval partial salpingectomy, and postpartum partial salpingectomy. The 5- and 10-year probabilities of pregnancy for the spring clip application were the least protective, with 31.7 pregnancies/1,000 procedures (95% CI 22.6 to 40.7) and 36.5 pregnancies/1,000 procedures (95% CI 25.3 to 47.7), respectively.

In contrast, unipolar coagulation and postpartum partial salpingectomy were the most protective, both with a 10-year probability of 7.5 pregnancies/1,000 procedures. When younger women 18 to 27 years undergo sterilization, they are at greater risk of conceiving than older women 33 to 44 years, 10 years after the initial procedure (Table 11-2). This increased risk is because of the increased inherent fertility of youth (increased ovarian reserve) and a longer interval for conception secondary to a longer exposure to sperm.

Although female sterilization is a highly effective method of contraception, women need to be counseled that failure rates are higher than previously reported. Some women using the Mirena® Intrauterine System (IUS) reported a 5-year cumulative failure rate of 7 pregnancies/1,000 women,[3] which is lower than all methods of female tubal sterilization procedures, which have a 5-year cumulative failure rate of 13.1 (95% CI 10.8 to 15.4). Individually, the Mirena® IUS has a lower failure rate than bipolar coagulation, silicone rubber band application, spring clip application, and interval partial salpingectomy (Table 11-1). Women who are ambivalent about sterilization may benefit from using the Mirena® IUS because it is removable.

Laparoscopic Interval Sterilization

Coagulation Procedures—Unipolar and Bipolar

Laparoscopic interval sterilization procedures are inherently more invasive and are associated with more morbidity and possible mortality.[4] In a review of deaths associated with female sterilization procedures performed in the United States between 1977 and 1981, 4 of 29 were likely attributable to the method of sterilization. Three of the four were caused by sepsis after apparent bowel injury during unipolar coagulation. Tissue coagulation occurs when electrons from an electrosurgical generator pass through tissue and desiccate it as heat accumulates. Coagulation continues until the resistance within the tissue does not allow any additional electric current to pass through. In unipolar coagulation, current passes from the operating instrument through the tissue to a grounding

Table 11-1: Life-Table Cumulative Probability of Pregnancy After Tubal Sterilization by Method

Method	Five Years After Sterilization/ 1,000 Procedures and 95% Confidence Interval (CI)
Bipolar coagulation	16.5 (10.6-22.4)
Unipolar coagulation	2.3 (0-4.8)
Silicone rubber band application	10 (6.4-13.5)
Spring clip application	31.7 (22.6-40.7)
Interval partial salpingectomy	15.1 (3.1-27.1)
Postpartum partial salpingectomy	6.3 (2.2-10.3)
All methods	13.1 (10.8-15.4)

Modified from Peterson et al[2]

plate attached to the patient. If the laparoscope is close to the grasping forceps (eg, an operating laparoscope), it could burn the bowel inadvertently, or electric current could pass through the bowel on its way to the grounding plate.[5] The desiccation of the fallopian tube that occurs from unipolar coagulation is more extensive than that from bipolar coagulation, which contributes to its low rate of sterilization failure. In both unipolar and bipolar coagulation, a portion of the isthmic segment of each fallopian tube is cauterized. In bipolar coagulation, one jaw of the

Ten Years After Sterilization/ 1,000 Procedures and 95% CI
24.8 (16.2-33.3)
7.5 (1.1-13.9)
17.7 (10.1-25.3)
36.5 (25.3-47.7)
20.1 (4.7-35.6)
7.5 (2.7-12.3)
18.5 (15.1-21.8)

grasping forceps is the active electrode, and the other jaw is the ground electrode. Low-voltage current is passed from one jaw of the forceps (active) through the tissue to the other jaw (ground). If resistance to the electric current builds up within the tissue, there may be incomplete desiccation. The larger the portion of tube desiccated (2 to 3 cm), the lesser the chance of sterilization failure. Upon healing, the cauterized portion of the tube will be absent, and a separation between the occluded proximal and distal ends of the cauterized area will exist.

Table 11-2: Life-Table Cumulative Probability of Pregnancy 10 Years After Tubal Sterilization (per 1,000 Procedures and 95% Confidence Interval) by Method and by Age at Sterilization

Sterilization Method	Age 18-27 Years
Bipolar coagulation	54.3 (28.3-80.4)
Unipolar coagulation	3.7 (0-11.1)
Silicone rubber band application	33.2 (10.6-55.9)
Spring clip application	52.1 (31-73.3)
Interval partial salpingectomy	9.7 (0-28.6)
Postpartum partial salpingectomy	11.4 (1.6-21.1)

Modified from Peterson et al[4]

Silicone Rubber Band Application

At laparoscopy, a silastic rubber band, often called a Falope-Ring® or Yoon ring, can be applied to a loop of the isthmic segment of the fallopian tube. Silastic is a mixture of silicone rubber, vulcanizing agents, and other additives. The silastic ring can be stretched to 6 mm for a few minutes while it is positioned over a grasped portion of the fallopian tube that is drawn into the inner cylinder of the silastic ring applicator. The silastic ring is then moved over the loop of tube and occludes the knuckle of tube. The distal loop is avascular because of the tight silastic band. After the distal end of the loop undergoes necrosis, the tube will be occluded and sometimes the proximal and

Age 34-44 Years
6.3 (0.1-12.5)
1.8 (0-5.3)
4.5 (0.6-8.4)
18.2 (0-36.4)
18.7 (0-39.6)
3.8 (0-11.4)

distal ends of the loop separate, leaving a space where tubal necrosis occurred.

Bleeding from mesosalpinx blood vessels or inadvertent laceration of the fallopian tube can be controlled with bipolar cautery. Patients should be informed that a coagulation procedure might have to be performed if there is bleeding or if the silastic band cannot be placed over a loop of tube because of adhesions or preexisting tubal dilation.

Spring Clip Application

At laparoscopy, the Hulka-Clemens spring clip can be applied to the isthmic portion of the fallopian tube. After the open clip is placed 90° to the long axis of the tube, it is applied with a laparoscopic introducer. The tube should rest against the hinge of the clip. After the clip is closed, a spring is pushed over the jaws of the clip to keep them closed. The Hulka-Clemens spring clip should also occlude a portion of the mesosalpinx. The tube is occluded and the two ends may separate, leaving a space where tubal necrosis occurred.

A modified version of the Hulka-Clemens spring clip is the longer Filshie clip. The Filshie clip is composed of titanium lined with silicone rubber. The US Food and Drug Administration (FDA) approved the Filshie clip in 1996. For application, this hinged clip is positioned over the isthmic segment with a special clip applicator. When the clip is closed, the silicone rubber expands to occlude the tube.

Because both the Hulka-Clemens and Filshie clips are narrow, only a small portion (approximately 5 mm) of the fallopian tube is damaged. This type of sterilization has the best chance of reversal by an anastomosis procedure to restore tubal patency.[6]

Interval Partial Salpingectomy

An interval partial salpingectomy can be performed either laparoscopically or via a laparotomy incision. Women who undergo sterilization through a laparotomy incision must be inherently more difficult to sterilize than with a laparoscopic procedure because of adhesions and/or tubal distortion. Women with the risk factors of obesity, prior pelvic infections, or previous surgery are more likely to have complications after sterilization through a laparotomy incision.[7]

Frequently Asked Question

If a Falope-Ring® falls off during initial placement, does it need to be retrieved?

A Falope-Ring® is inert and does not need to be retrieved.

Intrapartum and Postpartum Sterilization

Pomeroy Tubal Ligation

The Pomeroy tubal ligation was first described in 1929. It can be performed at the time of cesarean section or in the immediate postpartum period (<72 hours after delivery). In this procedure, the isthmic portion of the fallopian tube is elevated to form a loop, and a suture of plain catgut is used to ligate the base of the loop of tube. The knuckle of tube is excised. After healing, the catgut suture dissolves and the ends of the tube separate, leaving a space where the isthmic tube was excised.

Irving Tubal Ligation

The Irving tubal ligation was first described in 1924. It is usually performed at the time of cesarean section. The isthmic portion of the tube is excised, and the distal stump is ligated and buried within the broad ligament. The proximal end is ligated and buried in the fundus of the uterus.

Uchida Tubal Ligation

The Uchida tubal ligation was first described in 1946. It is usually performed at the time of cesarean section. The mesenteric portion of the tube is injected with saline. The isthmic portion of the tube is excised, and the distal end is occluded and left external to the broad ligament. The proximal end is ligated and buried within the broad ligament.

Frequently Asked Question

I'm having an emergency cesarean for fetal distress. I was scheduled to have a tubal ligation after this delivery. Should I still have a tubal ligation?

Depending on the status of the delivered infant, a woman might choose to delay her tubal ligation until the baby's health is assured. The delivering physician may be able to assess the infant's status shortly after delivery, before the abdomen is closed. If the infant's status is in doubt, a delay in performing the tubal ligation may be the most prudent choice. The physician should discuss this possibility with the mother if emergency delivery appears necessary.

Hysteroscopic Interval Sterilization

Essure® System (Conceptus Inc., San Carlos, CA)
www.essure.com
Toll-free telephone number:
1- 877-Essure1 (1-877-377-8731)

The Essure® System comprises the Essure® microinsert, a disposable delivery system, and a disposable split introducer. The Essure® microinsert is the actual device that is placed within the proximal segments of the tube, spanning the uterotubal junction. It is inserted in a wound-down configuration and allowed to expand when released from the introducer.

The Essure® microinsert has three components—a flexible stainless steel inner coil, a dynamic nickel titanium (Nitinol) expanding outer coil, and polyethylene terephthalate (PET) fibers. The PET fibers are wound in and around the inner coil. In its wound-down state, it is 4 cm long and 0.8 mm in diameter. When expanded, the outer coil is 1.5 to 2 mm in diameter and anchors the Essure® microinsert spanning the uterotubal junction into the proximal isthmic portion of the tube. After placement, there is a local tissue response that results in a chronic inflammatory and fibrotic response to the PET fibers. The local tissue in-growth against the PET aids in device retention and prevention of pregnancy.

The Essure® System is designed to be inserted in an outpatient setting with local or intravenous medication. A hysteroscopy is necessary, and, depending on individual characteristics, the patient may need a more formal, hospital operating room setting with general anesthesia. The perceived advantages for the patient are the absence of incisions, avoidance of intubation, and rapid recovery.

After the procedure, the patient is instructed that she is not protected from conception until a follow-up hysterosalpingogram (HSG) documents tubal occlusion. Women who are hypersensitive or allergic to nickel as confirmed by skin testing should not use Essure® microinserts. Women who are hypersensitive to radiographic contrast, precluding the follow-up HSG procedure, are also suboptimal candidates for this sterilization technique.

Contraceptive Efficacy

In a study of 518 previously fertile women, microinsert placement was attempted in 507 women and no placement was attempted in 11 women.[8] Bilateral placement of the microinserts was achieved in 446 women in the first attempt and in 18 women in the second. In total, bilateral placement of the microinserts was achieved in 92% (464/507) of the women. Three months after placement, 456 of the 464 women with bilateral microinsert placement underwent a HSG, and eight were not evaluated. The microinserts were satisfactorily located in 96% (437/456), and there was bilateral tubal occlusion in 92% (421/456). Of the 16 women who did not have tubal occlusion at 3 months, all had it by a follow-up HSG at 6 months after the sterilization procedure. Nine additional women with initial microinsert expulsion underwent a second placement procedure. All had successful placement and occlusion at 3 months verified by a HSG.

11

In summary, of the 456 women with bilateral microinsert placement and a follow-up HSG, 446 (98%) had bilateral tubal occlusion. As of January 2003, there were no pregnancies in this group of sterilized patients during 9,620 woman-months of observation and an average of 21.4 months of follow-up. In this study, 14 of the 20 investigators had no prior experience with the microinsert, and there was a wide range of expertise with hysteroscopic procedures. Future studies will need to examine the long-term, 5- to 10-year contraceptive efficacy rates among physicians inserting the microinserts.

Insertion of the Essure® Microinsert

Conceptus Inc., the manufacturer of the Essure® System, conducts medical education programs on the background and insertion of the Essure® microinsert. The program consists of a didactic portion and training with an Essure® placement simulator, followed by training with a preceptor. More information is available on the company's Web site www.conceptus.com or by telephone at 1-650-962-4060.

A brief summary of the insertion technique is as follows:

1. The insertion procedure should be performed in the follicular phase of the menstrual cycle to facilitate visualization of the fallopian tube ostia. When possible, the procedure should be performed on days 7 to 14 of the menstrual cycle.
2. A negative urine pregnancy test should be obtained on the day before the procedure.
3. Preoperative nonsteroidal anti-inflammatory medication should be administered 30 to 60 minutes before the procedure. Use of nonsteroidal anti-inflammatory medication has been associated with an increased placement success rate (odds ratio [OR]=2.6, 95% CI 1.1 to 5.8).[8]
4. For the insertion procedure, most women will require a paracervical block with a local anesthetic or intravenous medication for analgesia.
5. The microinsert is delivered by a system that fits through a 5-Fr (1.7-mm internal diameter) operative channel of a 5-mm outer diameter hysteroscope. When possible, dilation of the cervix is avoided.
6. With physiologic saline running to distend the cervix and provide forward vision for safe introduction of the hysteroscope, the uterus is inspected to document a normal cavity and identify the two tubal ostia. Standard monitoring of saline infusion for uterine distension should be observed during the procedure.

7. The microinsert should be inserted to a depth through the ostium so that 5 to 10 mm of its proximal end is visible at the ostium. To decrease the incidence of spontaneous expulsion, microinserts should be removed at the time of placement if 18 or more coils are visible in the uterine cavity.
8. After insertion of the two microinserts, patients should be observed postoperatively.

In the large study by Cooper et al,[8] the average procedure time was 36 minutes, and total time from entry to discharge from the recovery room was 80 minutes. Recovery was unremarkable in 58% (N=316) of procedures. In the remaining 228 procedures, the three most common symptoms were cramping (30%), pain (13%), and nausea (9%). Overall, 65% of participants (N=338) rated the pain associated with the insertion procedure as mild or none. Only 4% (N=21) rated the pain as severe. To ensure tubal occlusion, a HSG should be obtained 12 weeks after the procedure to document device location and the absence of tubal patency. Before the HSG, the patient should use an alternate form of reliable contraception.

Side Effects and Potential Complications of the Essure® System

In addition to the standard side effects of a hysteroscopy under either local anesthesia or intravenous medication, the major adverse events reported in the study by Cooper and colleagues[8] were expulsion of the microinsert (3%, N=14) and uterine perforation (0.9%, N=4). Expulsion of the microinsert occurs when an insufficient amount of it is placed within the tubal ostium. Uterine perforation can occur more often when there is poor identification of the tubal ostium or when preexisting tubal occlusion is present.

11

Women requesting the placement of Essure® microinserts should consider this sterilization procedure as permanent and irreversible. It is not known what the effect of the proximal intrauterine coils might have on endometrial development or a transferred embryo after in vitro fertilization. The coils could potentially be excised with hysteroscopic stainless steel microscissors, but the presence of the coils within the ostia may still have some unknown effect.[9]

Frequently Asked Question

I had an elective abortion 4 weeks ago. I'd like to consider Essure® microinserts. Do I need to wait a specific period before I can have the insertion procedure?

After any pregnancy (first-trimester abortion to term gestation), women should wait at least 6 weeks before inserting Essure® microinserts. Until spontaneous menstrual cycles return, they should use a reversible form of contraception before the placement of Essure® microinserts. Women should consider the decision for sterilization carefully and not make any decision while under physical or emotional stress.

References

1. Piccinino LJ, Mosher WD: Trends in contraceptive use in the United States: 1982-1995. *Fam Plann Perspect* 1998;30:4-10, 46.

2. Peterson HB, Xia Z, Hughes JM, et al: The risk of pregnancy after tubal sterilization: Findings from the U.S. Collaborative Review of Sterilization. *Am J Obstet Gynecol* 1996;174:1161-1170.

3. Mirena package insert. Berlex Laboratories, Monteville, NJ, 2003.

4. Peterson HB, DeStefano F, Rubin GL, et al: Deaths attributable to tubal sterilization in the United States, 1977-1981. *Am J Obstet Gynecol* 1983;146:131-136.

5. Centers for Disease Control and Prevention: Deaths following female sterilization with unipolar electrocoagulating devices. *MMWR* 1981;30:150.

6. Siegler AM, Hulka J, Peretz A: Reversibility of female sterilization. *Fertil Steril* 1985;43:499-510.

7. Layde PM, Peterson HB, Dicker RC, et al: Risk factors for complications of interval tubal sterilization by laparotomy. *Obstet Gynecol* 1983;62:180-184.

8. Cooper JM, Carignan CS, Cher D, et al: Microinsert nonincisional hysteroscopic sterilization. *Obstet Gynecol* 2003;102:59-67.

9. Ubeda A, Labastida R, Dexeus S: Essure: a new device for hysteroscopic tubal sterilization in an outpatient setting. *Fertil Steril* 2004;82:196-199.

Chapter 12

Male Sterilization

Vasectomy

When a couple considers the options for permanent sterilization, the multiple advantages of vasectomy exceed those of any female sterilization procedure. A vasectomy is a simple and safe office procedure and has few failures.[1] In a 1998 report of trends in contraceptive use from 1982 to 1995, 11% of reproductive-age women had partners with a vasectomy as their primary method of birth control.[2]

Traditional Vasectomy

In the traditional vasectomy procedure, the scrotum is anesthetized with a local anesthetic, 1% lidocaine without epinephrine. The health-care provider uses a scalpel to incise the scrotum once, or twice if a separate incision is needed for the second vas deferens. After the vas deferens is located, it is tied with a suture or occluded with a surgical clip and divided.[3] A portion of the vas deferens may be excised. Failure after suture ligation is likely caused by ischemic necrosis and sloughing of the vasal ends. The cut edges of the vas deferens are sometimes cauterized by a process called luminal fulguration. This process entails inserting a needle-tip cautery 3 to 4 mm into the vas lumen and withdrawing it slowly. This technique does not cause necrosis, but creates scarring and occlusion of the lumen. After both vas deferens are occluded, the skin incision is closed with a suture.

No-Scalpel Vasectomy

The traditional vasectomy procedure has undergone some refinement, and the no-scalpel vasectomy (NSV) technique uses a smaller incision to promote a faster recovery time, fewer complications, and potentially less discomfort.[4] In the NSV, the scrotum is anesthetized with a local anesthetic. The vas deferens is palpated and grasped with a ringed extracutaneous vas clamp, a special forceps used to fixate the vas deferens to the overlying skin. The medial blade of a dissecting forceps is used to pierce the scrotum, often in the midline or over one of the vas deferens. Once the scrotum is entered, a small loop of the vas deferens is elevated through the puncture or a small incision. A portion of the vas deferens is excised with cautery or suture ligated and removed. Sections of the vas deferens can be submitted for pathologic examination or held in storage and examined later, if an early failure occurs. The cut edges of the vas deferens are sometimes cauterized if suture ligated. The second vas deferens may be elevated through the same incision or a second incision. Because the skin incision can be a small puncture, it does not need to be closed with a suture.

Other Vasectomy Techniques

Other techniques have been used to occlude the vas deferens. One variation of the traditional vasectomy is to apply a titanium or plastic clip (VasClip®) to the vas deferens. The VasClip® is a locking, biocompatible, polymeric ligation band that can close the vas deferens in an atraumatic fashion.[5] The closed VasClip® is the size of a grain of rice. There is no randomized study to compare clip application with the NSV. Some health-care providers have cut the vas deferens with a laser and promoted this as a laser vasectomy. There are no benefits in using a laser to transect the vas deferens. Referrals to local health-care providers that perform the different vasectomy procedures can be found at the general Web site www.vasectomy.com.

Side Effects and Complications

The recovery period after a vasectomy is only a few days, with few complications. Some common side effects are pain and swelling of the scrotum with bruising, bleeding, or infection around the incision. Applying an ice pack to the scrotum decreases swelling. Limiting a patient's activity to sitting or reclining, rather than ambulating, in combination with oral analgesics will further help to relieve these symptoms. If walking is necessary, wearing tighter underwear briefs may provide better support to the scrotum than loose-fitting boxer shorts. The patient should be told to keep the scrotum dry and monitor for signs of an infection of the incision. In a review of complications of vasectomy, Raspa[6] reported bleeding or hematoma formation (1.6% to 4.6%) and incision infections (2.2% to 6%). Within the first year after a vasectomy, some men may develop an infrequent mild condition of epididymitis and orchitis (0.4% to 6.1%), a local inflammation of the epididymis and testis, which is responsive to heat therapy. Some sperm may also leak from the cut edge of the vas deferens, forming a small sperm granuloma (15% to 40%), which usually subsides spontaneously.

Contraceptive Efficacy

Men can resume sexual activity and ejaculate 3 to 4 days after the vasectomy. Men should be counseled that the interval to azoospermic semen samples varies, and that a certain number of ejaculations are necessary to deplete the remaining sperm in the male reproductive tract distal to the obstruction. During this period, alternate forms of contraception are necessary. Twelve weeks after the vasectomy, approximately 60% of men are azoospermic.[7] Men should have two azoospermic semen samples a month apart before they are informed they are sterilized. The failure rate from a vasectomy procedure is rare after persistent azoospermia is confirmed. In a study by Kaplan and Huether,[8] physicians with a high rate of success removed a significantly longer section of the vas deferens than did physicians with a low rate of success. The excised segments should be at least 15 mm in length. Segments shorter than 15 mm were associated with increased rates of recanalization. The actual failure rate from a vasectomy procedure appears to vary by the method of vas occlusion and the techniques used.[1] In the US Collaborative Review of Sterilization (CREST) study,[9] a group of 573 women whose husbands had vasectomies served as CREST controls. The cumulative probability of pregnancy in this group was 9.2/1,000 procedures at 1 year and 18.7/1,000 procedures at 2 years and remained constant through 5 years postvasectomy.[10] No information is available on the vasectomy method used in failures.

Men should consider vasectomy as permanent and only reversible with considerable effort and financial cost. Although a vasovasostomy procedure can be performed, the anastomosis of vas deferens is less likely when epididymal obstruction is present.[1] With the development of the fine-needle aspiration technique, testicular sperm aspiration allows men to have their sperm aspirated directly from the testicle under conscious sedation or a local anesthetic and not attempt to reverse their sterilization procedure.[11] Because of the small number of sperm retrieved, however, a single sperm must be directly injected into the oocyte by a process called intracytoplasmic sperm injection (ICSI). The ICSI procedure is performed in combination with controlled ovarian hyperstimulation of the woman for in vitro fertilization. For men with a failed vasovasostomy who do not wish to have a genetically linked child, insemination of the man's partner with donor semen is the procedure of choice.

Concept of Dual Methods

Vasectomy does not offer protection against the human immunodeficiency virus (HIV) or other sexually transmitted diseases (STDs). To protect themselves and their partners from these pathogens, vasectomized men should continue to use condoms.

Frequently Asked Question

After a vasectomy, will the force (velocity) or the volume of my ejaculate decrease?

Semen is the mixture of fluid ejaculated from various sources, including sperm. Because the prostate, seminal vesicles, and bulbourethral glands produce the most semen and semen is added after (distal) vas deferens occlusion, there is no perceived change in the volume or the velocity of semen ejaculated. Only a small amount of the fluid containing the sperm is derived from the testicle that is connected to the outflow tract by the vas deferens, which is now occluded by the vasectomy procedure.

References

1. Peterson HB, Huber DH, Belker AM, et al: Vasectomy: an appraisal for the obstetrician-gynecologist. *Obstet Gynecol* 1990;76:568.

2. Piccinino LJ, Mosher WD: Trends in contraceptive use in the United States: 1982-1995. *Fam Plann Perspect* 1998;30:4-10,46.

3. Reynolds RD: Vas deferens occlusion during no-scalpel vasectomy. *J Fam Pract* 1994;39:577-582.

4. Schlegal PN, Goldstein M: No-scalpel vasectomy. *Semin Urol* 1992;10:252-256.

5. VasClip® (Web page). VMBC, LLC, Web site. Available at: http://www.vasclip.com. Accessed March 2, 2007.

6. Raspa RF: Complications of vasectomy. *Am Fam Physician* 1993;48:1264-1268.

7. Barone MA, Nazerali H, Cortez M, et al: A prospective study of time and number of ejaculations to azoospermia after vasectomy by ligation and excision. *J Urol* 2003:170:892-896.

8. Kaplan KA, Huether CA: A clinical study of vasectomy failure and recanalization. *J Urol* 1975;113:71-74.

9. Peterson HB, Xia Z, Hughes JM, et al: The risk of pregnancy after tubal sterilization: findings from the US Collaborative Review of Sterilization. *Am J Obstet Gynecol* 1996;174:1161-1170.

10. Costello C: Pregnancies after Male or Female Sterilization. In: Sokal DC, ed: *Expert Consultation on Vasectomy Effectiveness.* Co-sponsored by Family Health International and Engender-

Health; April 18-19, 2001, Durham, NC. Available at: http://www.fhi.org/en/rh/pubs/booksreports/vasec_effective.htm. Accessed March 2, 2007.

11. Belker AM, Sherins RJ, Dennison-Lagos L, et al: Percutaneous testicular sperm aspiration: a convenient and effective office procedure to retrieve sperm for in vitro fertilization with intracytoplasmic sperm injection. *J Urol* 1998;160:2058-2062.

Chapter 13

Future Methods and Areas of Investigation

Implants: Progestin-Based

Norplant II

Norplant II is similar to the recently discontinued Norplant® System, but it consists of only two slightly larger rods rather than the six implants in the initial system. The US Food and Drug Administration (FDA) has approved Norplant II as a 3-year contraceptive, but it has not been introduced into the consumer market. Plans were to launch this version of the Norplant® System under the new trade name of Jadelle®. However, because of the adverse public response to the original Norplant® System, Norplant II may not be introduced in the United States.

Anti-Progestin Medication

Mifepristone (RU-486)

Mifeprex®
(Danco Laboratories, LLC, New York, NY)
http://www.earlyoptionpill.com
Toll-free telephone number: 1-877-4 Early Option (1-877-432-7596)

Mifepristone, the antiprogestin also known as RU-486 or Mifeprex®, was approved for the termination of early pregnancy in September 2000. To prevent opponents of the medication from boycotting a company's other medical products, the Population Council granted exclusive rights to Danco Laboratories to manufacture, market, and distribute their only product mifepristone under the trade name of Mifeprex®. As of 2004, more than 200,000 women had used Mifeprex® for the termination of pregnancy less than 49 days from their last menstrual period.

Mifepristone is a glucocorticoid receptor antagonist that has an affinity for the glucocorticoid receptor that is three times greater than dexamethasone. Mifepristone also binds to the progesterone receptor five times greater than progesterone. Mifepristone has a 25% affinity for the testosterone receptor and does not bind to the estrogen or mineralocorticoid receptor. In blocking the progesterone receptor, mifepristone use leads to endometrial instability and sloughing. In a pivotal study, Spitz et al[1] reported a 92% (762/827) termination rate in pregnancies of ≤49 days' gestational age treated with 600 mg of mifepristone followed by 400 μg of misoprostol (Cytotec®) 2 days after the mifepristone. This study defined the guidelines for the optimal patient who might use mifepristone for an early termination of pregnancy.

Subsequent studies have lowered the dose of mifepristone and asked whether an alternate dose of prostaglandin should be given. In a study by Creinin et al,[2] a lower dose of mifepristone (100 mg) followed in 2 days with 800 μg of misoprostol administered vaginally was more effective than the 400 μg of oral misoprostol. This study suggested that 100 mg of mifepristone might be just as effective as 600 mg of mifepristone when coupled with 800 μg of misoprostol administered vaginally.

The use of mifepristone for contraception, however, has been less promising. In a pilot study using 10 mg of mifepristone weekly vs planned postcoital administration of 10 mg of mifepristone within 5 days of coitus, the trial was stopped prematurely because of a high number of conceptions in both groups.[3] There were three pregnancies in 56 woman-months in the 10 mg of mifepristone weekly group. There were also three pregnancies in 68 woman-months in the postcoital mifepristone group. In both regimens, the proportion of ovulatory cycles indicated by ovulatory progesterone levels was 45%. The use of mifepristone should be limited to its indication of early pregnancy termination in pregnancies ≤49 days from the last menstrual period.

References

1. Spitz IM, Bardin CW, Benton L, et al: Early pregnancy termination with mifepristone and misoprostol in the United States. *N Engl J Med* 1998;338:1241-1247.

2. Creinin MD, Pymar HC, Schwartz JL, et al: Mifepristone 100 mg in abortion regimens. *Obstet Gynecol* 2001;98:434-439.

3. Godfrey EM, Mawson JT, Stanwood NL, et al: Low-dose mifepristone for contraception: a weekly versus planned postcoital randomized pilot study. *Contraception* 2004;70:41-46.

Appendix A

Efficacy of Different Contraceptive Methods

Method	Perfect Use*	Typical Use*	Research Findings/ Comments
No method	85%	85%	—
Withdrawal method	4%	27%	23.6%**
Periodic abstinence		25%	20.5%**
Calendar	9%		
Standard Days Method™ (CycleBeads™)	4.75%[1]	11.96%[1]	
Spermicide	18%	29%	25.7%**
Conceptrol® 100 mg tablet			44%[2]
VCF® 72 mg			39.8%[2]

*Unless otherwise noted, data in these columns are 1-year probabilities of pregnancy. From Trussell J: Contraceptive efficacy. In: Hatcher RA, Trussell J, Stewart F, et al: *Contraceptive Technology*, 18th ed. New York, NY, Ardent Media, 2004, pp 778-845.
**Contraceptive failure rate corrected for abortion underreporting in an unstandardized group. Data from Fu et al, *Fam Plann Perspect* 1999;31:56-63.

Method	Perfect Use*	Typical Use*	Research Findings/ Comments
Condom (used without spermicide)			
Male	2%	15%	13.9%**
Female	5%	21%	
Cervical cap (used with spermicide)			12.1%** (combined with diaphragm use)
Nulliparous women	9%	16%	
Parous women	26%	32%	
FemCap™ cervical cap with spermicide			Package insert states: 23% (all sizes)*** 14% (22 mm) 14% (26 mm) 29% (30 mm)
Lea's Shield® with spermicide			5.6% [†,3] Package insert states: 15%***
Diaphragm (used with spermicide)	6%	16%	12.1%** (combined with cervical cap use)

*Unless otherwise noted, data in these columns are 1-year probabilities of pregnancy. From Trussell J: Contraceptive efficacy. In: Hatcher RA, Trussell J, Stewart F, et al: *Contraceptive Technology*, 18th ed. New York, NY, Ardent Media, 2004, pp 778-845.
**Contraceptive failure rate corrected for abortion underreporting in an unstandardized group. Data from Fu et al, *Fam Plann Perspect* 1999;31:56-63.

Method	Perfect Use*	Typical Use*	Research Findings/ Comments
Sponge			
Nulliparous women	9%	16%	
Parous women	20%	32%	
Oral contraceptive pills			
Combination	0.3%	8%	7.6%**
Progestin only	0.3%	8%	In typical use, PI=0.2[4] PI varies with age:[5] ≤40 years, PI=3.1 >40 years, PI=0.3
Contraceptive patch (Ortho Evra®)	0.3%	8%	PI varies with body weight:[6] ≤90 kg, PI=0.7 >90 kg, PI=6.0
Contraceptive ring (NuvaRing®)	0.3%	8%	PI=0.65[7]
Progestin injectable (DMPA)	0.3%	0.3%	3.1%**

**One-year probabilities are projected from 6-month study. Only 6-month pregnancy rate available.
DMPA=depot medroxyprogesterone acetate,
PI=Pearl Index (number of contraceptive failures/ 100 woman-years of exposure)

Method	Perfect Use*	Typical Use*	Research Findings/ Comments
Progestin implant	0.05%	0.05%	1.8%**
Intrauterine device			
Copper-T	0.6%	0.8%	
Levonorgestrel-releasing	0.1%	0.1%	
Female sterilization (tubal ligation)	0.5%	0.5%	
Vasectomy	0.1%	0.15%	

*Unless otherwise noted, data in these columns are 1-year probabilities of pregnancy. From Trussell J: Contraceptive efficacy. In: Hatcher RA, Trussell J, Stewart F, et al: *Contraceptive Technology*, 18th ed. New York, NY, Ardent Media, 2004, pp 778-845.
**Contraceptive failure rate corrected for abortion underreporting in an unstandardized group. Data from Fu et al, *Fam Plann Perspect* 1999;31:56-63.

References

1. Arévalo M, Jennings V, Sinai I: Efficacy of a new metho[d] of family planning: the Standard Days Method. *Contraceptio[n]* 2002;65:333-338.

2. Raymond E, Dominik R: Contraceptive effectiveness of tw[o] spermicides: a randomized trial. *Obstet Gynecol* 1999;93:896-903

3. Mauck C, Glover LH, Miller E, et al: Lea's Shield: a study o[f] the safety and efficacy of a new vaginal barrier contraceptive use[d] with and without spermicide. *Contraception* 1996;53:329-335.

4. Broome M, Fotherby K: Clinical experience with the progestogen-only pill. *Contraception* 1990;42:489-495.

5. Vessey MP, Lawless M, Yeates D, et al: Progestogen-only ora[l] contraception. Findings in a large prospective study with specia[l] reference to effectiveness. *Br J Fam Plann* 1985;10:117-121.

6. Zieman M, Guillebaud J, Weisberg E, et al: Contraceptive efficacy and cycle control with the Ortho Evra/Evra transdermal system: the analysis of pooled data. *Fertil Steril* 2002;77(2 suppl 2):S13-S18.

7. Roumen FJ, Apter D, Mulders TM, et al: Efficacy, tolerability and acceptability of a novel contraceptive vaginal ring releasing etonogestrel and ethinyl oestradiol. *Hum Reprod* 2001;16:469-475.

Appendix B

Oral Contraceptive Pills Listed Alphabetically

Brand Name*	Manufacturer
Alesse®	Wyeth
Apri®	Barr
Aviane®	Barr
Balziva™	Barr
Brevicon®	Watson
Camila®	Barr
Cryselle® 28	Barr
Cyclessa®	Organon
Demulen® 1/35**	Pfizer
Demulen® 1/50	Pfizer
Desogen®	Organon
Enpresse® 28	Barr
Errin®	Barr

*All oral contraceptive pills (OCPs) listed are available in the United States unless otherwise noted.

**Discontinued

Estrogen Dose (μg)	Progestin Dose (mg)
EE 20	LNG 0.100
EE 30	DSG 0.150
EE 20	LNG 0.100
EE 35	NET 0.4
EE 35	NET 0.5
—	NET 0.35
EE 30	NRG 0.300
EE 25	DSG 0.100, 7 days 0.125, 7 days 0.150, 7 days
EE 35	ETD 1.0
EE 50	ETD 1.0
EE 30	DSG 0.150
EE 30, 6 days EE 40, 5 days EE 30, 10 days	LNG 0.050, 6 days 0.075, 5 days 0.125, 10 days
—	NET 0.35

Brand Name*	Manufacturer
Estrostep® Fe	Warner Chilcott
Femcon® Fe	Warner Chilcott
Jenest®**	Organon
Jolivette®	Watson
Junel™ Fe 1/20	Barr
Junel™ Fe 1.5/30	Barr
Kariva®	Barr
Leena™	Watson
Lessina® 28	Barr
Levlen® 28	Berlex
Levlite®	Berlex
Levora® 0.15/30-28	Watson
Loestrin® 24 Fe	Warner Chilcott
Loestrin® Fe 1/20	Barr
Loestrin® Fe 1.5/30	Barr
Lo/Ovral®	Wyeth
Low-Ogestrel®	Watson
Lutera™	Watson
Microgestin® Fe 1/20	Watson
Microgestin® Fe 1.5/30	Watson

*All OCPs listed are available in the United States unless otherwise noted.

**Discontinued

Estrogen Dose (μg)	Progestin Dose (mg)
EE 20, 5 days 30, 7 days 35, 9 days	NETA 1.0
EE 35	NET 0.4
EE 35	NET 0.5, 7 days 1.0, 14 days
—	NET 0.35
EE 20	NETA 1.0
EE 30	NETA 1.5
EE 20	DSG 0.150
EE 35	NET 0.5, 7 days 1.0, 9 days 0.5, 5 days
EE 20	LNG 0.100
EE 30	LNG 0.150
EE 20	LNG 0.100
EE 30	LNG 0.150
EE 20	NETA 1.0
EE 20	NETA 1.0
EE 30	NETA 1.5
EE 30	NRG 0.300
EE 30	NRG 0.300
EE 20	LNG 0.100
EE 20	NETA 1.0
EE 30	NETA 1.5

Brand Name*	Manufacturer
Micronor®	Ortho-McNeil
Mircette®	Barr
Modicon®	Ortho-McNeil
MonoNessa®	Watson
Necon® 0.5/35	Watson
Necon® 1/35	Watson
Necon® 1/50	Watson
Necon® 7/7/7	Watson
Necon® 10/11	Watson
Nor-QD®	Watson
Nora-BE®	Watson
Nordette®	Monarch
Norinyl® 1+35	Watson
Norinyl® 1+50	Watson
Nortrel® 0.5/35	Barr
Nortrel® 1/35	Barr
Nortrel® 7/7/7	Barr
Ogestrel® 0.5/50	Watson
Ortho-Cept®	Ortho-McNeil
Ortho-Cyclen®	Ortho-McNeil

*All OCPs listed are available in the United States unless otherwise noted.

Estrogen Dose (μg)	Progestin Dose (mg)
—	NET 0.35
EE 20	DSG 0.150
EE 35	NET 0.5
EE 35	NGM 0.250
EE 35	NET 0.5
EE 35	NET 1.0
M 50	NET 1.0
EE 35	NET 0.5, 7 days 0.75, 7 days 1.0, 7 days
EE 35	NET 0.5, 10 days 1.0, 11 days
—	NET 0.35
—	NET 0.35
EE 30	LNG 0.150
EE 35	NET 1.0
M 50	NET 1.0
EE 35	NET 0.5
EE 35	NET 1.0
EE 35	NET 0.5, 7 days 0.75, 7 days 1.0, 7 days
EE 50	NRG 0.5
EE 30	DSG 0.150
EE 35	NGM 0.250

Brand Name*	Manufacturer
Ortho-Novum® 1/35	Ortho-McNeil
Ortho-Novum® 1/50	Ortho-McNeil
Ortho-Novum® 7/7/7	Ortho-McNeil
Ortho-Novum® 10/11	Ortho-McNeil
Ortho Tri-Cyclen®	Ortho-McNeil
Ortho Tri-Cyclen® Lo	Ortho-McNeil
Ovcon® 35	Warner Chilcott
Ovcon® 50	Warner Chilcott
Ovral®-28	Wyeth
Ovrette®	Wyeth
Portia® 28	Barr
Seasonale®	Barr
Seasonique™	Barr
Sprintec®	Barr
Tri-Levlen® 28	Berlex

*All OCPs listed are available in the United States unless otherwise noted.

Estrogen Dose (μg)	Progestin Dose (mg)
EE 35	NET 1.0
M 50	NET 1.0
EE 35	NET 0.5, 7 days 0.75, 7 days 1.0, 7 days
EE 35	NET 0.5, 10 days 1.0, 11 days
EE 35	NGM 0.180, 7 days 0.215, 7 days 0.250, 7 days
EE 25	NGM 0.180, 7 days 0.215, 7 days 0.250, 7 days
EE 35	NET 0.4
EE 50	NET 1.0
EE 50	NRG 0.500
—	NRG 0.075
EE 30	LNG 0.150
EE 30	LNG 0.150
EE 30	LNG 0.150
EE 35	NGM 0.250
EE 30, 6 days EE 40, 5 days EE 30, 10 days	LNG 0.050, 6 days 0.075, 5 days 0.125, 10 days

Brand Name*	**Manufacturer**
Tri-Norinyl®-28	Watson
Tri-Sprintec®	Barr
TriNessa®	Watson
Triphasil®-28	Wyeth
Trivora®-28	Watson
Velivet™	Barr
Yasmin®	Berlex
YAZ®	Berlex
Zovia® 1/35E	Watson
Zovia® 1/50E	Watson

*All oral contraceptive pills listed are available in the United States unless otherwise noted.

DSG = desogestrel
DRSP = drospirenone
EE = ethinyl estradiol
ETD = ethynodiol diacetate
LNG = levonorgestrel

Estrogen Dose (μg)	Progestin Dose (mg)
EE 35	NET 0.5, 7 days 1.0, 9 days 0.5, 5 days
EE 35	NGM 0.180, 7 days 0.215, 7 days 0.250, 7 days
EE 35	NGM 0.180, 7 days 0.215, 7 days 0.250, 7 days
EE 30, 6 days EE 40, 5 days EE 30, 10 days	LNG 0.050, 6 days 0.075, 5 days 0.125, 10 days
EE 30, 6 days EE 40, 5 days EE 30, 10 days	LNG 0.050, 6 days 0.075, 5 days 0.125, 10 days
EE 25	DSG 0.100, 7 days 0.125, 7 days 0.150, 7 days
EE 30	DRSP 3.0
EE 20	DRSP 3.0
EE 35	ETD 1.0
EE 50	ETD 1.0

M = mestranol
NET = norethindrone
NETA = norethindrone acetate
NGM = norgestimate
NRG = norgestrel

Appendix C

Oral Contraceptive Pills Listed by Manufacturer

Name	Estrogen Dose (μg)	Progestin Dose (mg)
Berlex Laboratories www.berlex.com		
Levlite®	EE 20	LNG 0.100
YAZ®	EE 20	DRSP 3.0
Levlen® 28	EE 30	LNG 0.150
Yasmin®	EE 30	DRSP 3.0
Tri-Levlen® 28	EE 30, 6 days EE 40, 5 days EE 30, 10 days	LNG 0.050, 6 days 0.075, 5 days 0.125, 10 days
Duramed Pharmaceuticals, Inc./ Barr Laboratories, Inc. www.barrlabs.com		
Camila®	—	NET 0.35
Errin®	—	NET 0.35
Loestrin® Fe 1/20	EE 20	NETA 1.0

Active Pill Color	Placebo Pill Color	Remarks
Pink	White	
Light pink	White	24 active pills, 4 inert placebo pills www.yaz-us.com
Light orange	Pink	Available as Levlen® 21 (21 active pills)
Yellow	White	www.yasmin.com
Brown White Light yellow	Light green	Available as Tri-Levlen® 21 (21 active pills)
Light pink	—	
Yellow	—	
White	Brown	7 ferrous fumarate, 75 mg, iron placebo pills, also available without iron; in Canada, pill is known as Minestrin® 1/20

Name	Estrogen Dose (µg)	Progestin Dose (mg)
Duramed Pharmaceuticals, Inc./ Barr Laboratories, Inc. *(continued)*		
Junel™ Fe 1/20	EE 20	NETA 1.0
Aviane®	EE 20	LNG 0.100
Lessina® 28	EE 20	LNG 0.100
Kariva®	EE 20	DSG 0.150
Mircette®	EE 20	DSG 0.150
Velivet™	EE 25	DSG 0.100, 7 days 0.125, 7 days 0.150, 7 days
Loestrin® Fe 1.5/30	EE 30	NETA 1.5
Junel™ Fe 1.5/30	EE 30	NETA 1.5
Cryselle® 28	EE 30	NRG 0.300
Portia® 28	EE 30	LNG 0.150
Seasonale®	EE 30	LNG 0.150

Active Pill Color	Placebo Pill Color	Remarks
Light yellow	Brown	7 ferrous fumarate, 75 mg, iron placebo pills, also available without iron
Orange	Light green	
Pink	White	
White	Light green	21 active pills, 2 placebos, 5 EE, 10 μg/pill (Light blue)
White	Green	21 active pills, 2 placebos, 5 EE, 10 μg/pill (yellow); www.mircette.com; also known as Mercilon® worldwide, but has 21 active and 7 placebo pills www.mircette.com
Beige Orange Pink	White	
Green	Brown	7 ferrous fumarate, 75 mg, iron placebo pills, also available without iron
Pink	Brown	7 ferrous fumarate, 75 mg, iron placebo pills, also available without iron
White	Light green	
Pink	White	
Pink	White	84 active pills, 7 placebos per pack, www.seasonale.com

Name	Estrogen Dose (μg)	Progestin Dose (mg)
Duramed Pharmaceuticals, Inc./ Barr Laboratories, Inc. *(continued)*		
Seasonique™	EE 30	LNG 0.150
Apri®	EE 30	DSG 0.150
Enpresse® 28	EE 30, 6 days EE 40, 5 days EE 30, 10 days	LNG 0.050, 6 days 0.075, 5 days 0.125, 10 days
Balziva™	EE 35	NET 0.4
Nortrel® 0.5/35	EE 35	NET 0.5
Nortrel® 1/35	EE 35	NET 1.0
Nortrel® 7/7/7	EE 35	NET 0.5, 7 days 0.75, 7 days 1.0, 7 days
Sprintec®	EE 35	NGM 0.250
Tri-Sprintec®	EE 35	NGM 0.180, 7 days 0.215, 7 days 0.250, 7 days
Monarch Pharmaceuticals www.kingpharm.com		
Nordette®	EE 30	LNG 0.150
Organon Inc. www.organon.com		
Cyclessa®	EE 25	DSG 0.100, 7 days 0.125, 7 days 0.150, 7 days

Active Pill Color	Placebo Pill Color	Remarks
Light blue-green	Yellow	84 active pills, 7 EE, 10 μg/pill www.seasonique.com
Rose	White	
Pink White Orange	Light green	
Light peach	White	Active pills not chewable.
Light yellow	White	
Yellow	White	
Light yellow Blue Peach	White	
Blue	White	
Gray Light blue Blue	White	
Light orange	Pink	
Light yellow Orange Red	Green	www.cyclessa.com

Name	Estrogen Dose (μg)	Progestin Dose (mg)
Ortho-McNeil Pharmaceutical www.orthowomenshealth.com		
Desogen®	EE 30	DSG 0.150
Jenest®	EE 35	NET 0.5, 7 days 1.0, 14 days
Micronor®	—	NET 0.35
Ortho Tri-Cyclen® Lo	EE 25	NGM 0.180, 7 days 0.215, 7 days 0.250, 7 days
Ortho-Cept®	EE 30	DSG 0.150
Modicon®	EE 35	NET 0.5
Ortho-Novum® 1/35	EE 35	NET 1.0
Ortho-Novum® 10/11	EE 35	NET 0.5, 10 days 1.0, 11 days
Ortho-Novum® 7/7/7	EE 35	NET 0.5, 7 days 0.75, 7 days 1.0, 7 days
Ortho-Cyclen®	EE 35	NGM 0.250
Ortho Tri-Cyclen®	EE 35	NGM 0.180, 7 days 0.215, 7 days 0.250, 7 days
Ortho-Novum® 1/50	M 50	NET 1.0

Active Pill Color	Placebo Pill Color	Remarks
White	Green	Also known as Marvelon® worldwide.
White Peach	Green	Discontinued
Lime green	—	
White Light blue Dark blue	Green	www.orthotri-cyclenlo.com
Orange	Green	
White	Green	
Peach	Green	
White Peach	Green	
White Light peach Peach	Green	
Blue	Green	
White Light blue Blue	Green	
Yellow	Green	

Name	Estrogen Dose (μg)	Progestin Dose (mg)
Pfizer Pharmaceuticals, Inc. www.pfizer.com		
Demulen® 1/35	EE 35	ETD 1.0
Demulen® 1/50	EE 50	ETD 1.0
Warner Chilcott www.wcrx.com		
Loestrin® 24 Fe	EE 20	NETA 1.0
Estrostep® Fe	EE 20, 5 days 30, 7 days 35, 9 days	NETA 1.0
Ovcon® 35	EE 35	NET 0.4
Femcon® Fe	EE 35	NET 0.4
Ovcon® 50	EE 50	NET 1.0
Watson Laboratories, Inc. www.watsonpharm.com		
Jolivette®	—	NET 0.35
Nora-BE®	—	NET 0.35
Nor-QD®	—	NET 0.35
Microgestin® Fe 1/20	EE 20	NETA 1.0

Active Pill Color	Placebo Pill Color	Remarks
White	Blue	Active pills do not contain lactose, placebo pills contain lactose; discontinued.
Pink	Blue	Active pills do not contain lactose, placebo pills contain lactose.
White	Brown	24 active pills, 4 ferrous fumarate, 75 mg, iron placebo pills www.shortperiod.com
White triangle White square White round	Brown	7 ferrous fumarate, 75 mg, iron placebo pills
Peach	White	
White	Brown	chewable active pills, 7 ferrous fumarate, 75 mg, iron placebo pills
Yellow	Green	
Lime green	—	
White	—	
Yellow	—	
White	Brown	7 ferrous fumarate, 75 mg, iron placebo pills, also available without iron.

Name	Estrogen Dose (μg)	Progestin Dose (mg)
Watson Laboratories, Inc. *(continued)*		
Lutera™	EE 20	LNG 0.100
Microgestin® Fe 1.5/30	EE 30	NETA 1.5
Levora® 0.15/20-28	EE 30	LNG 0.150
Low-Ogestrel®	EE 30	NRG 0.300
Brevicon®	EE 35	NET 0.5
Necon® 0.5/35	EE 35	NET 0.5
Norinyl® 1+35	EE 35	NET 1.0
Necon® 1/35	EE 35	NET 1.0
Zovia® 1/35E	EE 35	ETD 1.0
Trivora®-28	EE 30, 6 days EE 40, 5 days EE 30, 10 days	LNG 0.050, 6 days 0.075, 5 days 0.125, 10 days
Necon® 10/11	EE 35	NET 0.5, 10 days 1.0, 11 days
Necon® 7/7/7	EE 35	NET 0.5, 7 days 0.75, 7 days 1.0, 7 days
Tri-Norinyl®-28	EE 35	NET 0.5, 7 days 1.0, 9 days 0.5, 5 days
Leena™	EE 35	NET 0.5, 7 days 1.0, 9 days 0.5, 5 days
MonoNessa®	EE 35	NGM 0.250

Active Pill Color	Placebo Pill Color	Remarks
White	Peach	
Green	Brown	7 ferrous fumarate, 75 mg, iron placebo pills, also available without iron.
White	Peach	
White	Peach	
Blue	Orange	
Light yellow	White	
Yellow-green	Orange	
Dark yellow	White	
Light pink	White	
Blue White Pink	Peach	
Light yellow Dark yellow	White	
White Light peach Peach	Green	
Blue Yellow-green Blue	Orange	
Blue Yellow-green Blue	Orange	
Blue	Green	

Name	Estrogen Dose (μg)	Progestin Dose (mg)
Watson Laboratories, Inc. *(continued)*		
TriNessa®	EE 35	NGM 0.180, 7 days 0.215, 7 days 0.250, 7 days
Necon® 1/50	M 50	NET 1.0
Norinyl® 1+50	M 50	NET 1.0
Zovia® 1/50E	EE 50	ETD 1.0
Ogestrel® 0.5/50	EE 50	NRG 0.5
Wyeth **www.wyeth.com**		
Ovrette®	—	NRG 0.075
Alesse®	EE 20	LNG 0.100
Lo/Ovral®	EE 30	NRG 0.300
Triphasil®-28	EE 30, 6 days EE 40, 5 days EE 30, 10 days	LNG 0.050, 6 days 0.075, 5 days 0.125, 10 days
Ovral®-28	EE 50	NRG 0.500

Abbreviations

DSG = desogestrel
DRSP = drospirenone
EE = ethinyl estradiol
ETD = ethynodiol diacetate
LNG = levonorgestrel

Active Pill Color	Placebo Pill Color	Remarks
White Light blue Blue	Green	
Light blue	White	
White	Orange	
Pink	White	
White	Peach	
Yellow	—	
Pink	Green	
Brown White Light yellow	Light green	Available as Triphasil®-21 (21 active pills)
White	Pink	

M = mestranol
NET = norethindrone
NETA = norethindrone acetate
NGM = norgestimate
NRG = norgestrel

Appendix D

Oral Contraceptive Pills Listed by Dose and Formulation

Brand Name	Generic Product
Monophasic (listed by increasing estrogen dose)	
Loestrin® 24 Fe	———
Loestrin® Fe 1/20	Microgestin® Fe 1/20 Junel™ Fe 1/20
Alesse®	Aviane®
Levlite®	Lessina® 28 Lutera™
Mircette®	Kariva®
YAZ®	———
Loestrin® Fe 1.5/30	Microgestin® Fe 1.5/30 Junel™ Fe 1.5/30
Levlen®	Levora®
Nordette®	Portia® 28
Seasonale®	

Estrogen Dose (μg)	Progestin Dose (mg)	Remarks
EE 20	NETA 1.0	24 active pills, 4 iron placebo pills
EE 20	NETA 1.0	Also available as a 21-day pack without iron placebo pills.
EE 20	LNG 0.100	
EE 20	DSG 0.150	21 active pills, 2 placebo, 5 EE, 10 μg/pill
EE 20	DRSP 3.0	24 active pills, 4 inert placebo pills
EE 30	NETA 1.5	Also available as a 21-day pack without iron placebo pills.
EE 30	LNG 0.150	
EE 30	LNG 0.150	84 active pills, 7 placebos per pack

Brand Name	Generic Product
Monophasic (listed by increasing estrogen dose) *(continued)*	
Seasonique™	———
Desogen®, Ortho-Cept®	Apri®
Lo/Ovral®	Low-Ogestrel® Cryselle® 28
Yasmin®	
Ovcon® 35	Balziva™
Femcon® Fe	———
Modicon®	Necon® 0.5/35
Brevicon®	Nortrel® 0.5/35
Ortho-Novum® 1/35	Necon® 1/35
Norinyl® 1+35	Nortrel® 1/35
Demulen® 1/35	Zovia® 1/35E
Ortho-Cyclen®	Sprintec® MonoNessa®
Ortho-Novum® 1/50, Norinyl® 1+50	Necon® 1/50
Ovcon® 50	
Demulen® 1/50	Zovia® 1/50E
Ovral®-28	Ogestrel®

Estrogen Dose (μg)	Progestin Dose (mg)	Remarks
EE 30	LNG 0.150	84 active pills, 7 EE 10 μg/pill
EE 30	DSG 0.150	
EE 30	NRG 0.300	
EE 30	DRSP 3.0	
EE 35	NET 0.4	Active pills not chewable, inert placebo pills.
EE 35	NET 0.4	Chewable active pills, 7 iron placebo pills
EE 35	NET 0.5	
EE 35	NET 1.0	
EE 35	ETD 1.0	Discontinued
EE 35	NGM 0.250	
M 50	NET 1.0	
EE 50	NET 1.0	
EE 50	ETD 1.0	
EE 50	NRG 0.5	

Brand Name	Generic Product
Multiphasic (listed by increasing estrogen dose)	
Estrostep® Fe	
Cyclessa®	Velivet™
Ortho Tri-Cyclen® Lo	
Ortho-Novum® 10/11	Necon® 10/11
Jenest®	
Ortho-Novum® 7/7/7	Nortrel® 7/7/7 Necon® 7/7/7
Tri-Norinyl®-28	Leena™
Ortho Tri-Cyclen®	Tri-Sprintec® TriNessa®
Tri-Levlen® 28	Trivora®-28
Triphasil®-28	Enpresse® 28

Estrogen Dose (μg)	Progestin Dose (mg)	Remarks
EE 20, 5 days EE 30, 7 days EE 35, 9 days	NETA 1.0	
EE 25	DSG 0.100, 7 days 0.125, 7 days 0.150, 7 days	
EE 25	NGM 0.180, 7 days 0.215, 7 days 0.250, 7 days	
EE 35	NET 0.5, 10 days 1.0, 11 days	
EE 35	NET 0.5, 7 days 1.0, 14 days	Discontinued
EE 35	NET 0.5, 7 days 0.75, 7 days 1.0, 7 days	
EE 35	NET 0.5, 7 days 1.0, 9 days 0.5, 5 days	
EE 35	NGM 0.180, 7 days 0.215, 7 days 0.250, 7 days	
EE 30, 6 days	LNG 0.050, 6 days	
EE 40, 5 days EE 30, 10 days	0.075, 5 days 0.125, 10 days	

Brand Name	Generic Product
Progestin-only Pills	
Micronor®	Errin® Jolivette® Nora-BE®
Nor-QD®	Camila®
Ovrette®	

DSG = desogestrel
DRSP = drospirenone
EE = ethinyl estradiol
ETD = ethynodiol diacetate
LNG = levonorgestrel

Estrogen Dose (μg)	Progestin Dose (mg)	Remarks
—	NET 0.35	
—	NET 0.35	
—	NRG 0.075	

M = mestranol
NET = norethindrone
NETA = norethindrone acetate
NGM = norgestimate
NRG = norgestrel

Index

C

D

E

I

J

K

L

M

N

O

R

S

T

Y

Z

Contemporary Guide to Contraception™

Retail $22.50

Ordering Information

Prices (in U.S. dollars)

1 book:	$22.50 each
2-9 books:	$20.25 each
10-99 books:	$18.00 each
> 99 books:	Call 800-860-9544*

How to Order:

1. by telephone: 800-860-9544*
2. by fax: 215-860-9558
3. by Internet: www.HHCbooks.com
4. by mail: Handbooks in Health Care Co.
   3 Terry Drive, Suite 201
   Newtown, PA 18940

Shipping/Handling

Books will be shipped via Priority Mail or UPS Ground unless otherwise requested.

1-3 books:	$6.00
4-9 books:	$8.00
10-14 books:	$11.00
15-24 books:	$13.00
> 24 books:	Plus shipping

International orders: Please inquire

*Please call between 9 AM and 5 PM EST Monday through Friday, 800-860-9544.

Pennsylvania residents must add 6% sales tax.

Prices good through November 30, 2008

Color Atlas of Oral Contraceptive Pills

The following color atlas of oral contraceptive pills is presented to identify, illustrate, and clarify each individual product. The pictures are presented by order of increasing estrogen dose and then by increasing generation of the progestin compound. A sincere effort was made to purchase or obtain samples of each product to photograph in a uniform fashion. When pills were not available to purchase, manufacturers were contacted to obtain samples, but not all manufacturers supplied samples. For completeness, two recently discontinued pills (Jenest® and Demulen® 1/35) are listed in Appendix D, but they are not pictured in the atlas. One pill (Ovrette®) was not available from the manufacturer to photograph and was not available to purchase.

Section A: Monophasic

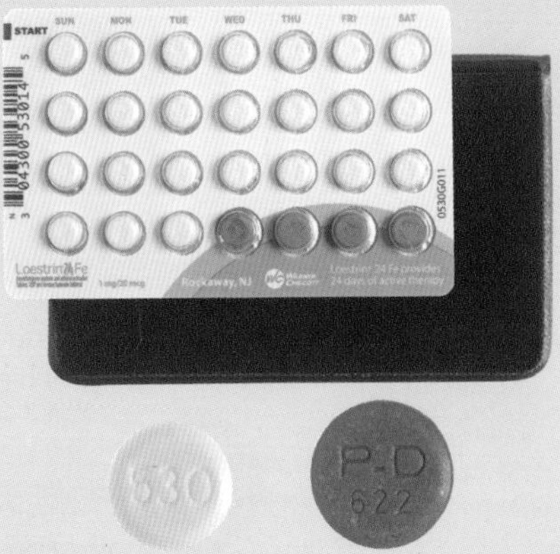

Loestrin® 24 Fe
(ethinyl estradiol/norethindrone acetate)

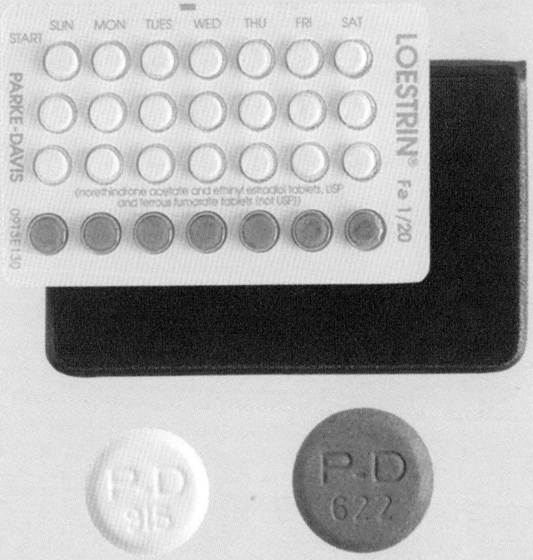

Loestrin® Fe 1/20
(ethinyl estradiol/norethindrone acetate)

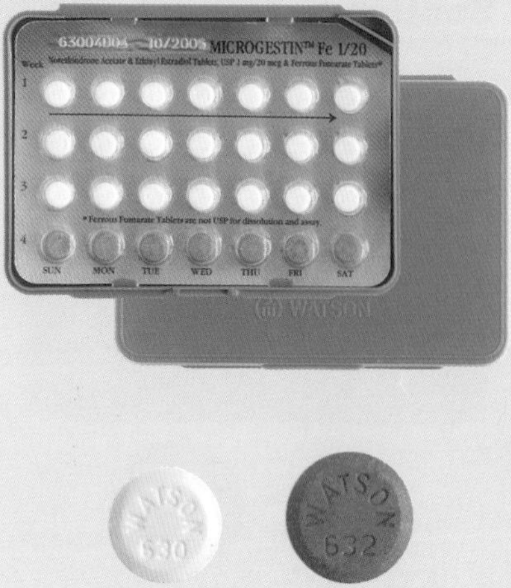

Microgestin® Fe 1/20
(ethinyl estradiol/norethindrone acetate)

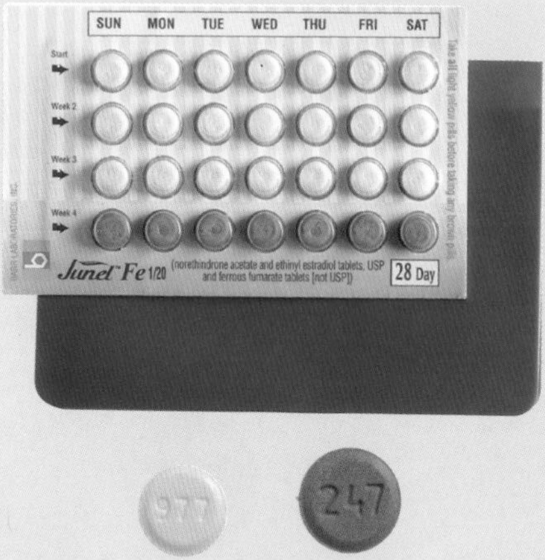

Junel™ Fe 1/20
(ethinyl estradiol/norethindrone acetate)

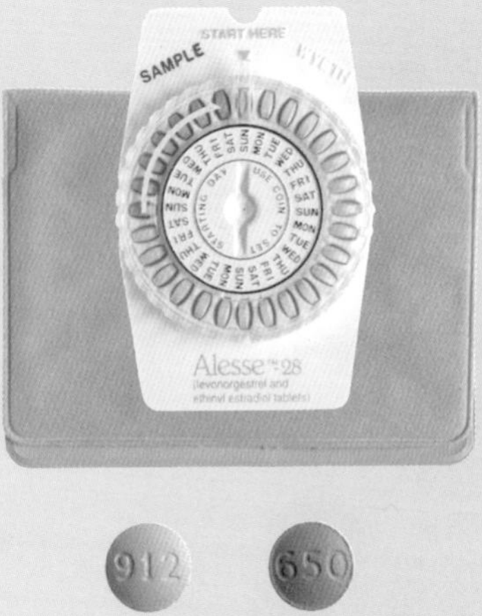

Alesse®
(ethinyl estradiol/levonorgestrel)

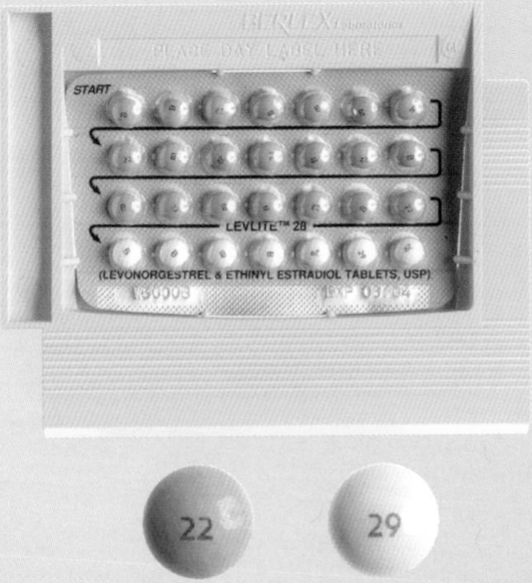

Levlite®
(ethinyl estradiol/levonorgestrel)

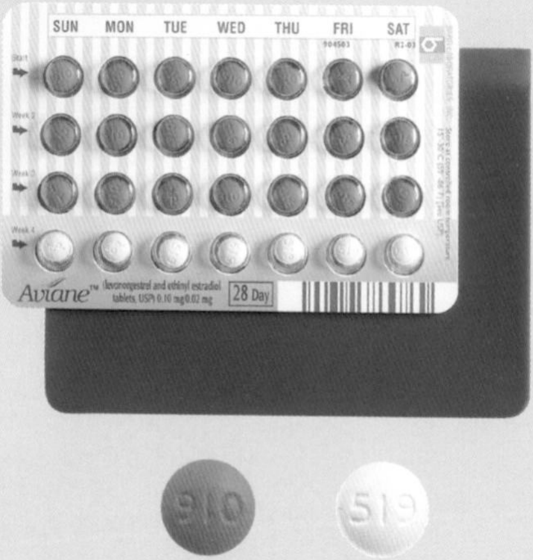

Aviane®
(ethinyl estradiol/levonorgestrel)

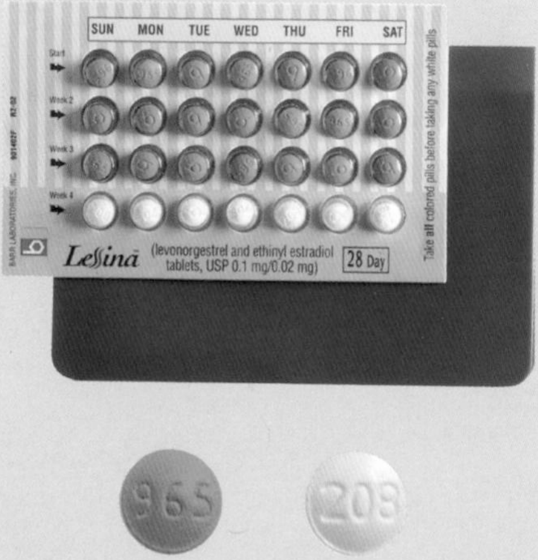

Lessina® 28
(ethinyl estradiol/levonorgestrel)

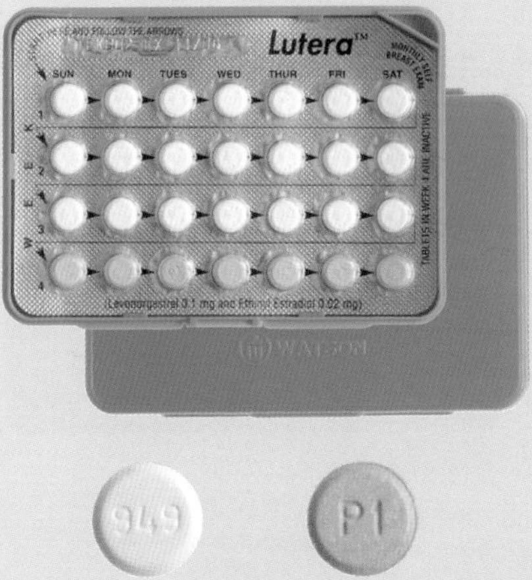

Lutera™
(ethinyl estradiol/levonorgestrel)

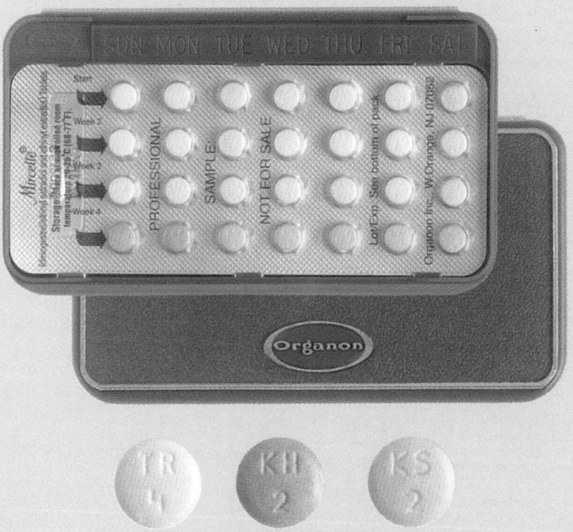

Mircette®
(ethinyl estradiol/desogestrel)

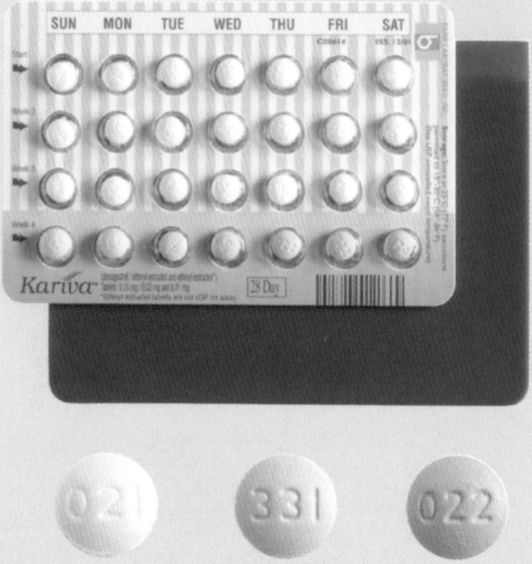

Kariva®
(ethinyl estradiol/desogestrel)

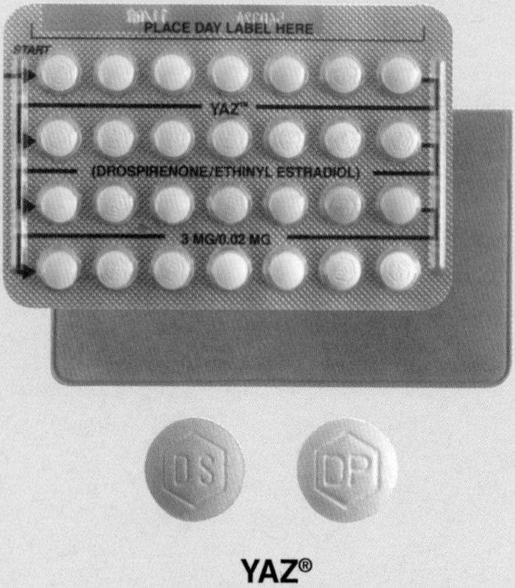

YAZ®
(ethinyl estradiol/drospirenone)

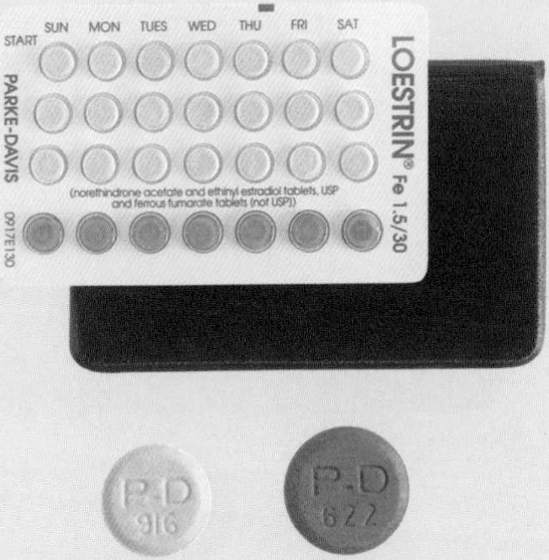

Loestrin® Fe 1.5/30
(ethinyl estradiol/norethindrone acetate)

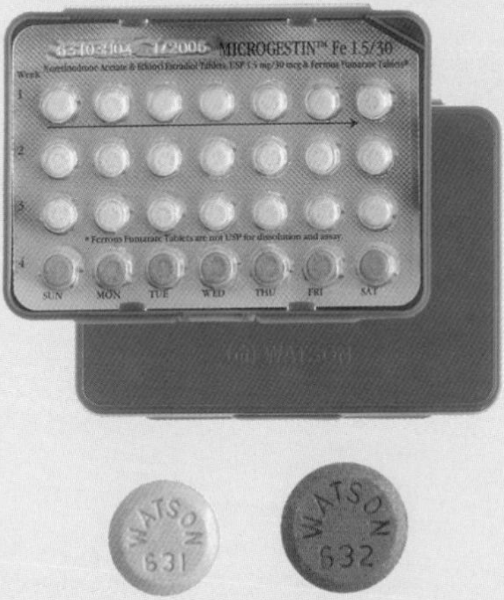

Microgestin® Fe 1.5/30
(ethinyl estradiol/norethindrone acetate)

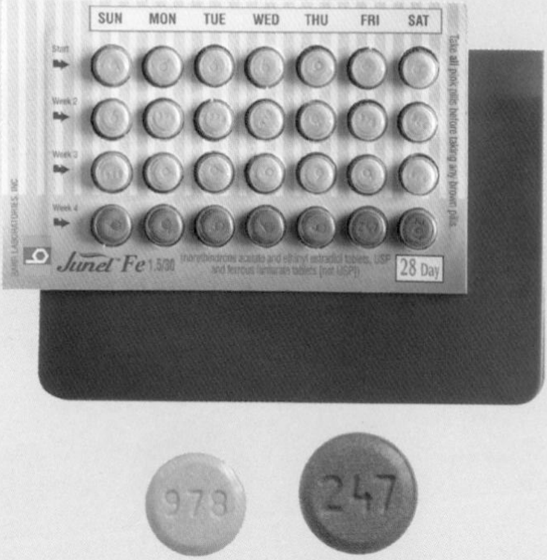

Junel™ Fe 1.5/30
(ethinyl estradiol/norethindrone acetate)

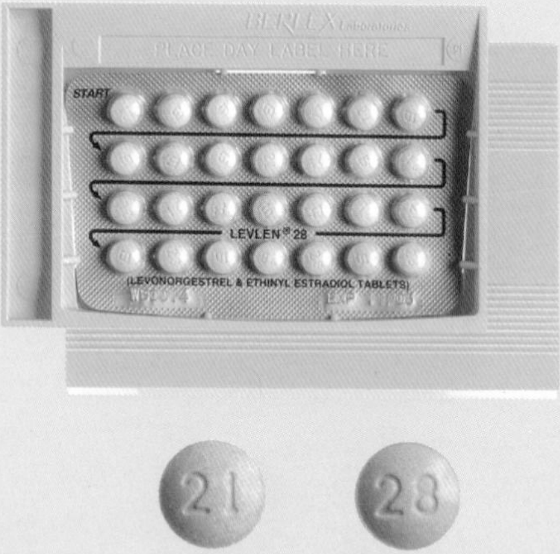

Levlen®
(ethinyl estradiol/levonorgestrel)

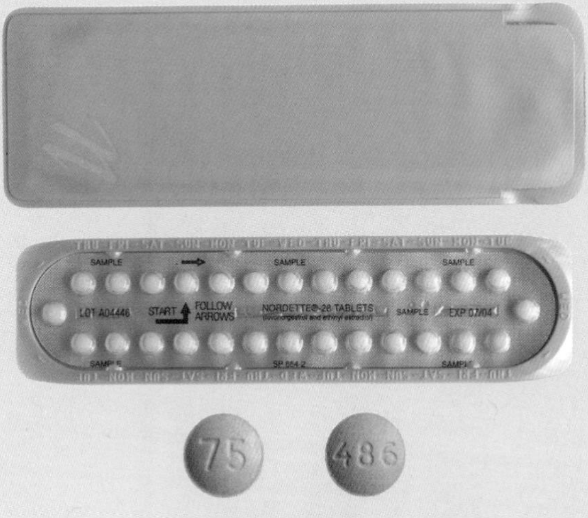

Nordette®
(ethinyl estradiol/levonorgestrel)

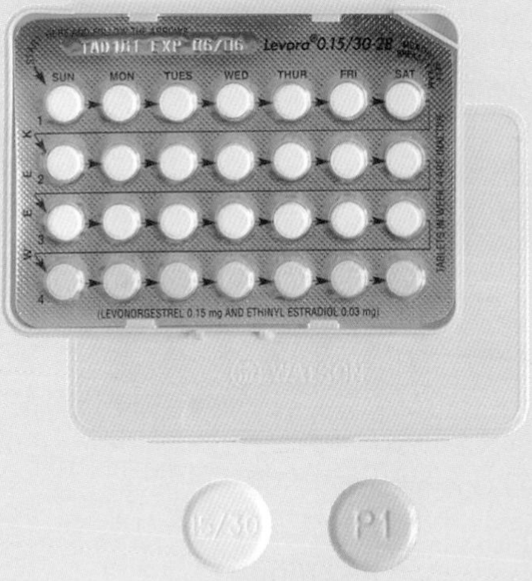

Levora®
(ethinyl estradiol/levonorgestrel)

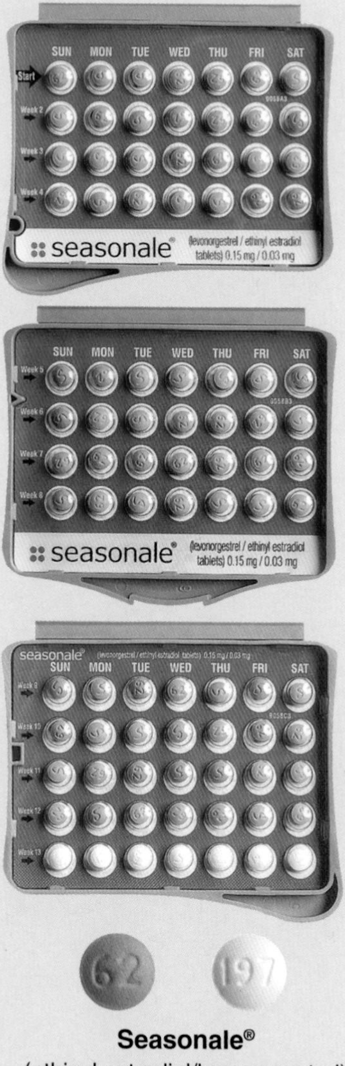

Seasonale®

(ethinyl estradiol/levonorgestrel)

Continued on next page

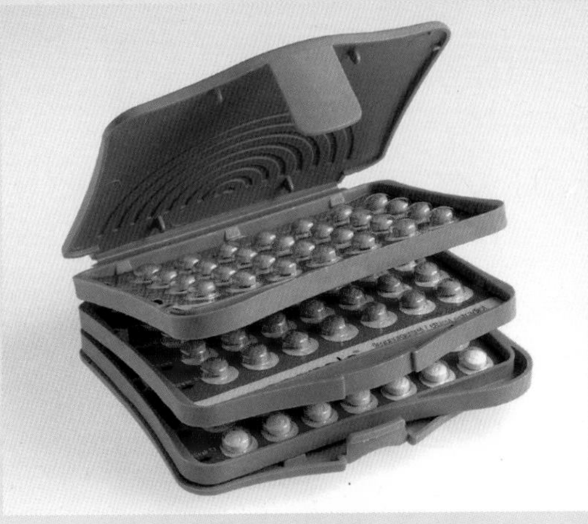

Seasonale®
(ethinyl estradiol/levonorgestrel)

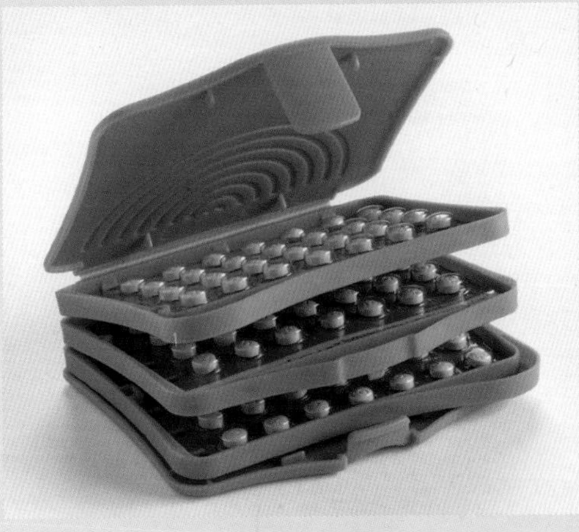

Seasonique™
(ethinyl estradiol/levonorgestrel)
Continued on next page

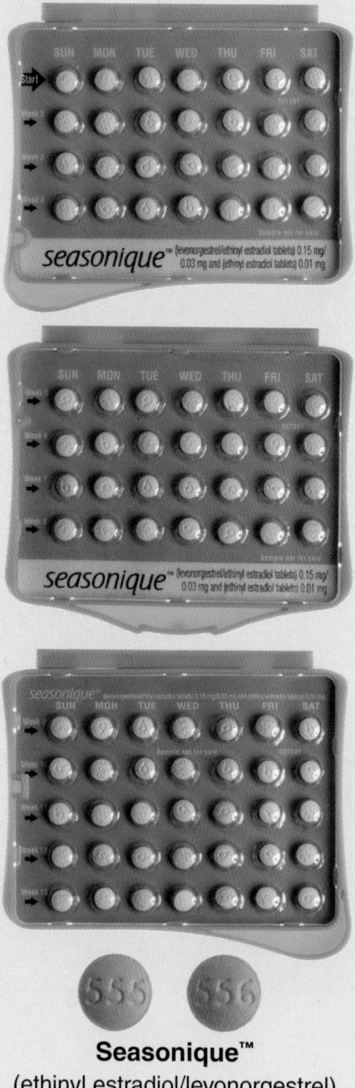

Seasonique™

(ethinyl estradiol/levonorgestrel)

Continued from page A-11

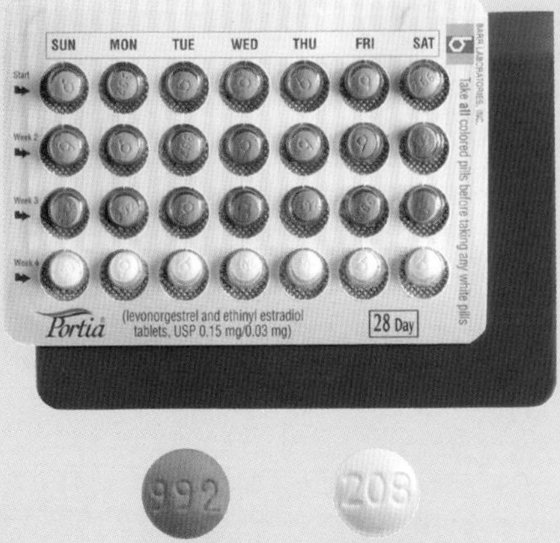

Portia® 28
(ethinyl estradiol/levonorgestrel)

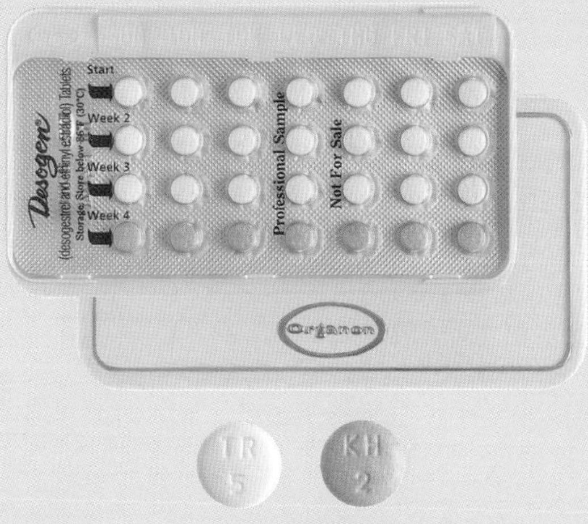

Desogen®
(ethinyl estradiol/desogestrel)

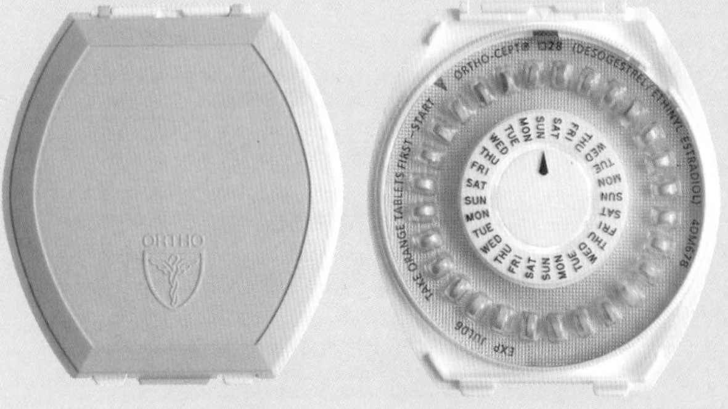

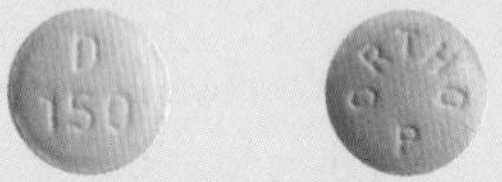

Ortho-Cept®
(ethinyl estradiol/desogestrel)

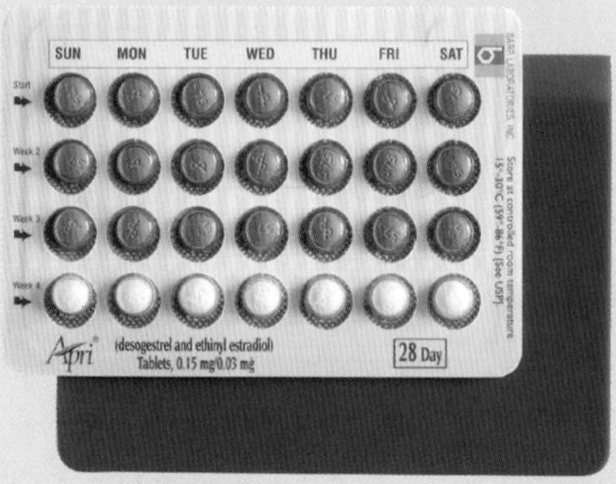

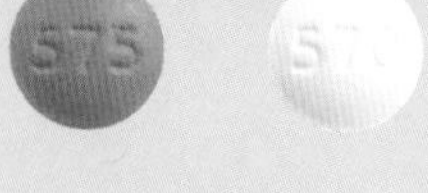

Apri®
(ethinyl estradiol/desogestrel)

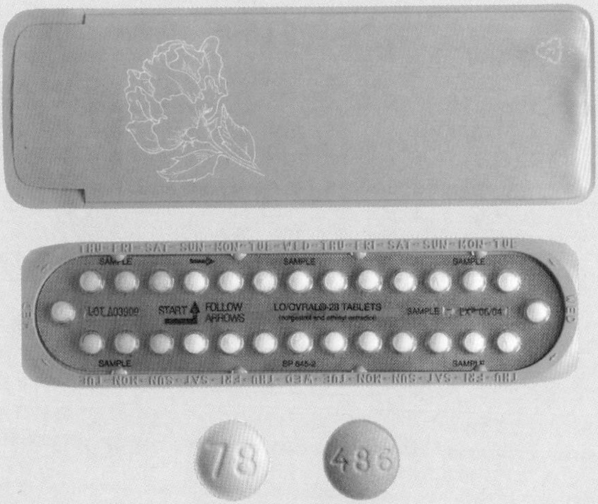

Lo/Ovral®

(ethinyl estradiol/norgestrel)

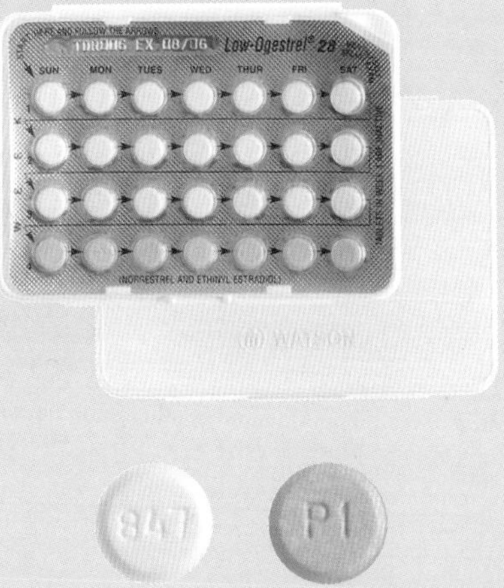

Low-Ogestrel®

(ethinyl estradiol/norgestrel)

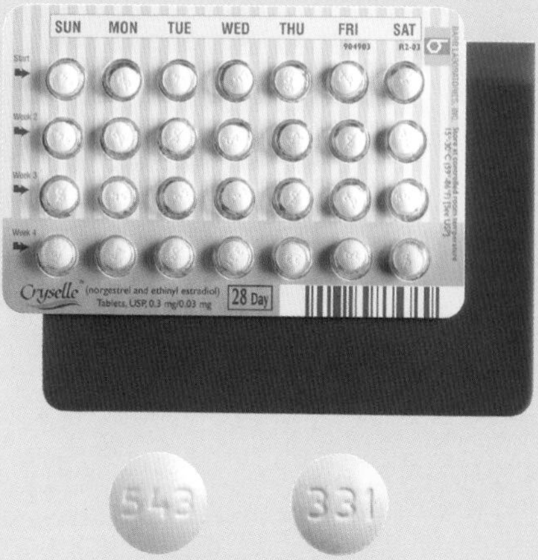

Cryselle® 28
(ethinyl estradiol/norgestrel)

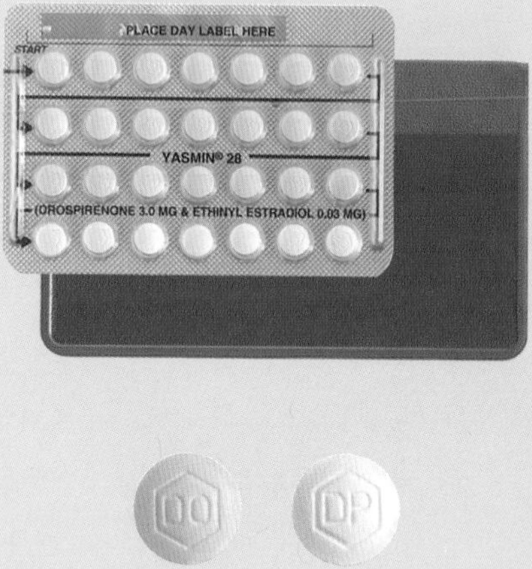

Yasmin®
(ethinyl estradiol/drospirenone)

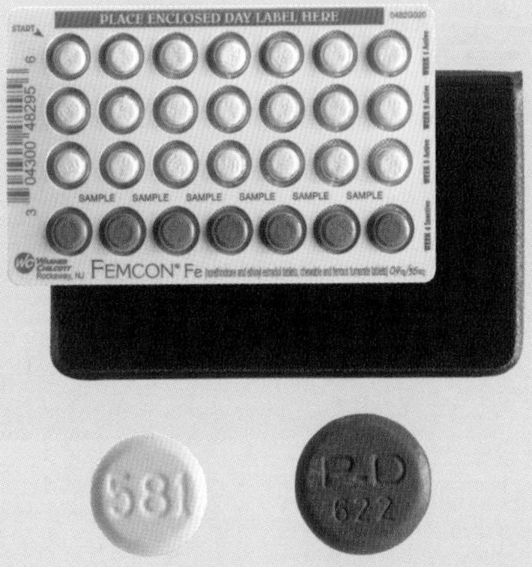

Femcon® Fe
(ethinyl estradiol/norethindrone)

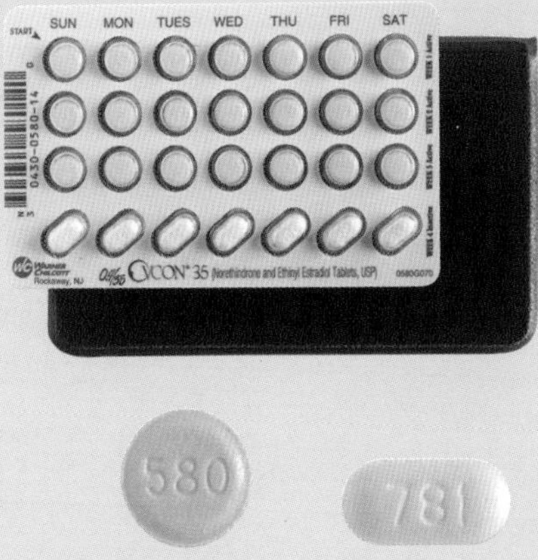

Ovcon® 35
(ethinyl estradiol/norethindrone)

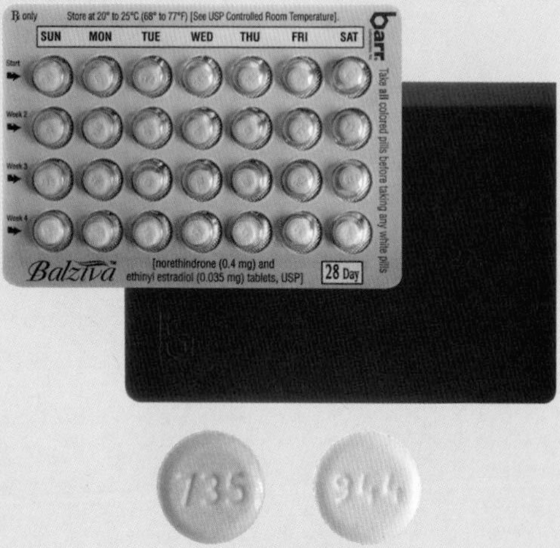

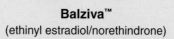

Balziva™
(ethinyl estradiol/norethindrone)

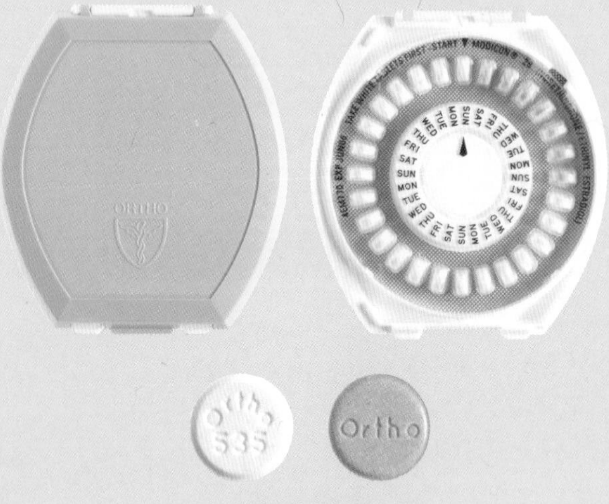

Modicon®
(ethinyl estradiol/norethindrone)

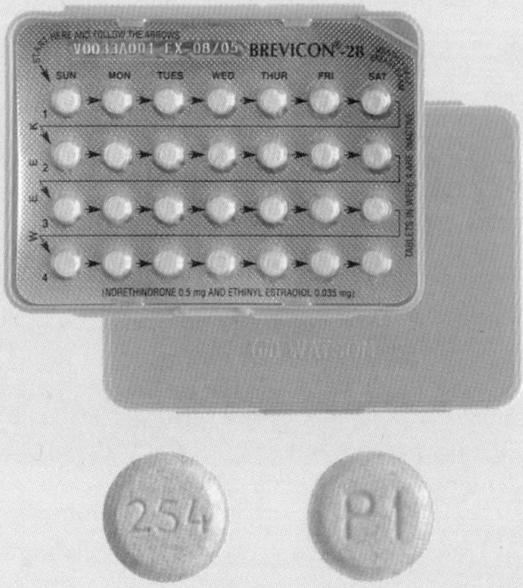

Brevicon®
(ethinyl estradiol/norethindrone)

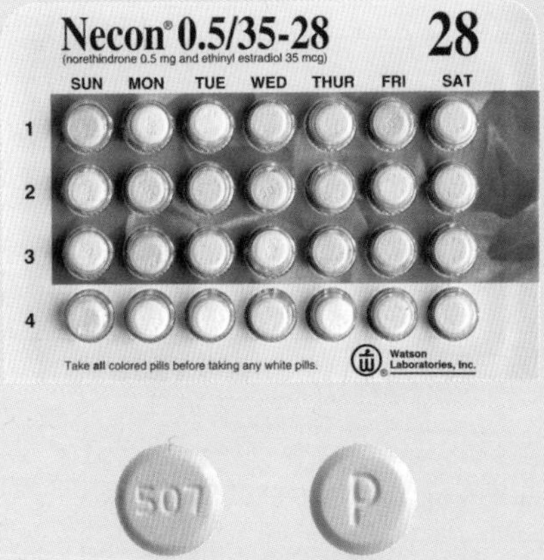

Necon® 0.5/35
(ethinyl estradiol/norethindrone)

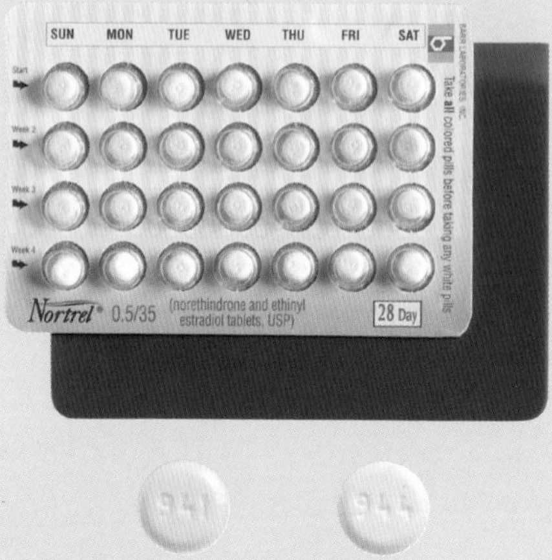

Nortrel® 0.5/35
(ethinyl estradiol/norethindrone)

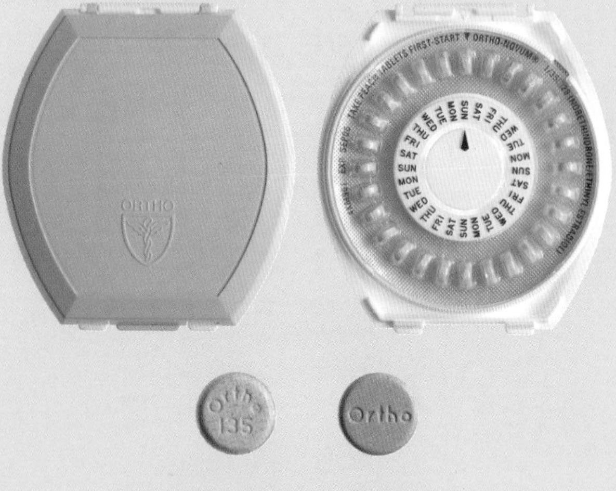

Ortho-Novum® 1/35
(ethinyl estradiol/norethindrone)

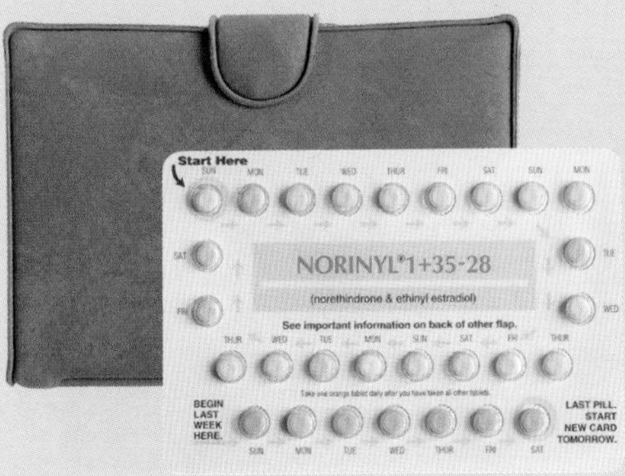

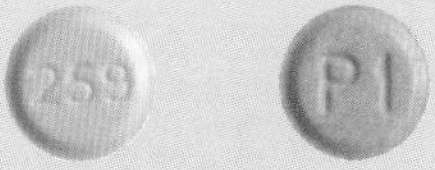

Norinyl® 1+35
(ethinyl estradiol/norethindrone)

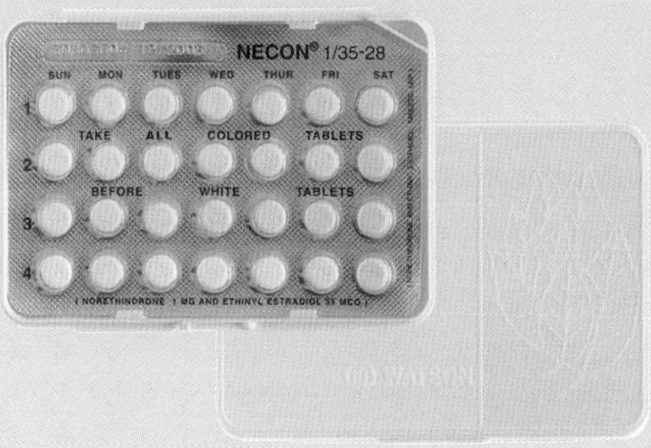

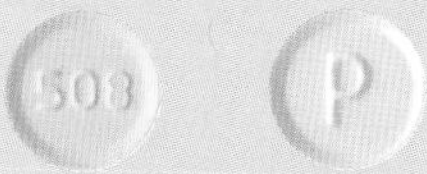

Necon® 1/35
(ethinyl estradiol/norethindrone)

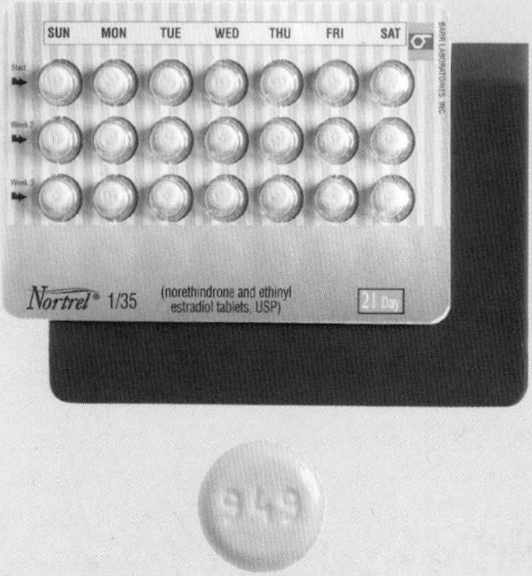

Nortrel® 1/35
(ethinyl estradiol/norethindrone)

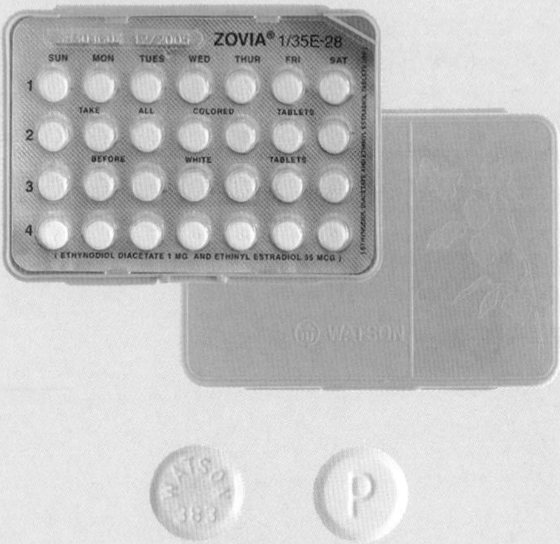

Zovia® 1/35E
(ethinyl estradiol/ethynodiol diacetate)

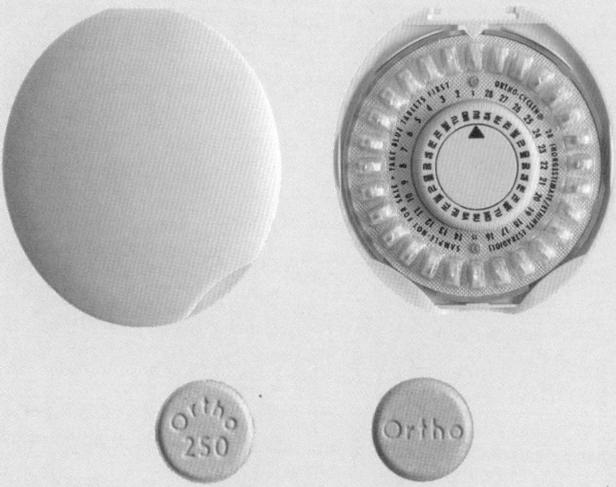

Ortho-Cyclen®
(ethinyl estradiol/norgestimate)

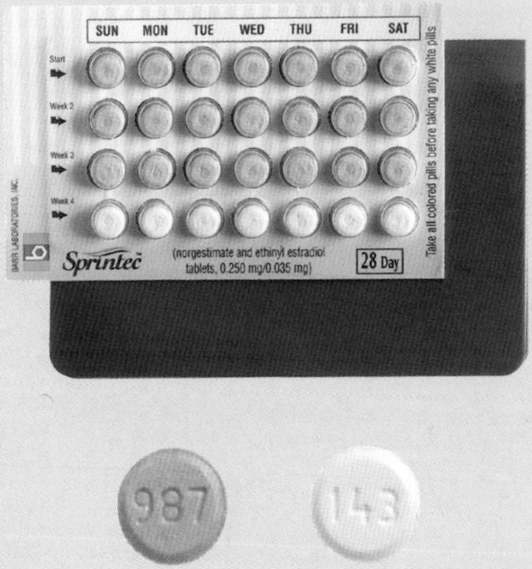

Sprintec®
(ethinyl estradiol/norgestimate)

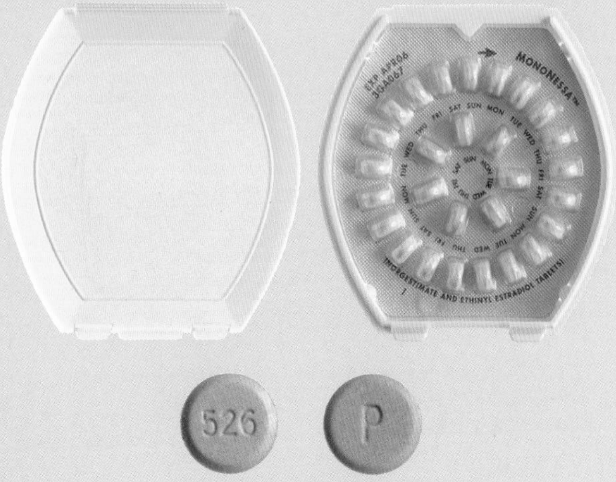

MonoNessa®
(ethinyl estradiol/norgestimate)

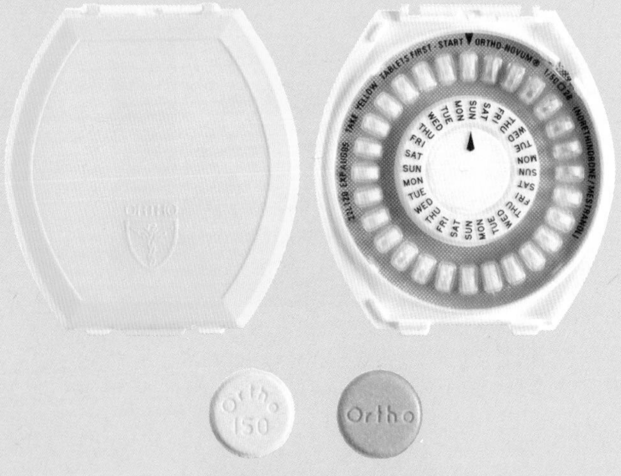

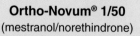

Ortho-Novum® 1/50
(mestranol/norethindrone)

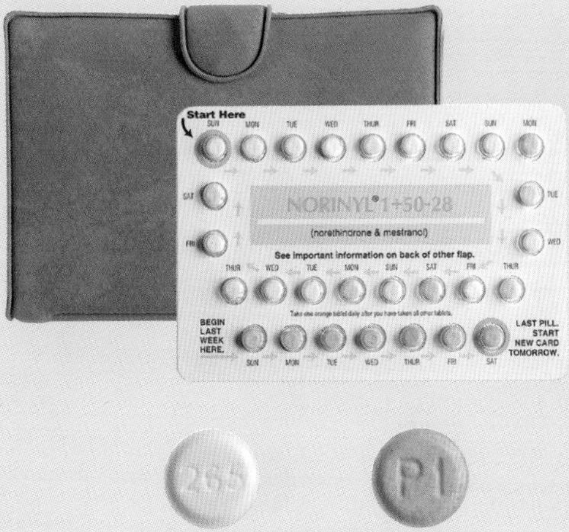

Norinyl® 1+50
(mestranol/norethindrone)

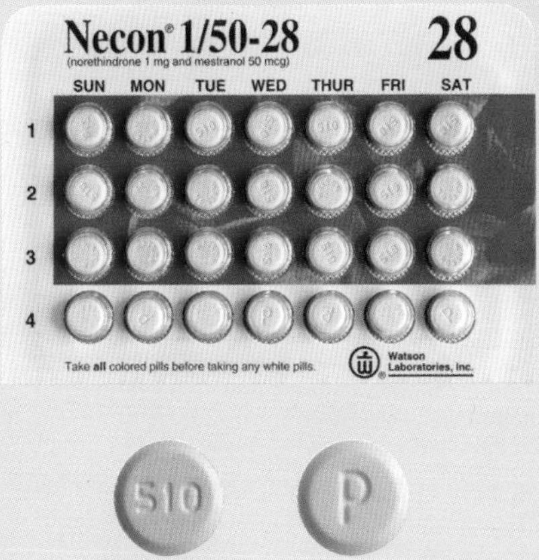

Necon® 1/50
(mestranol/norethindrone)

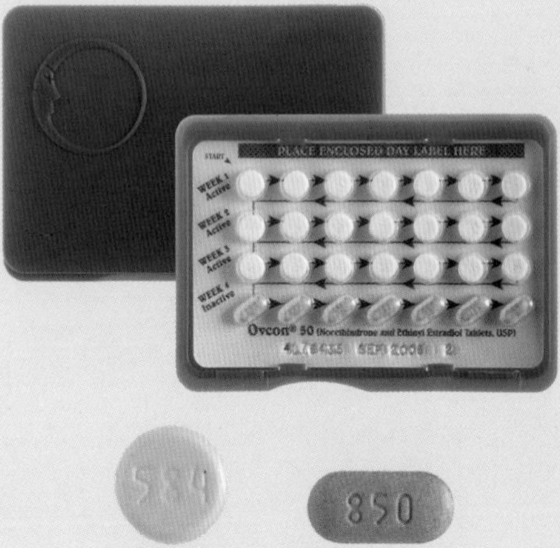

Ovcon® 50
(ethinyl estradiol/norethindrone)

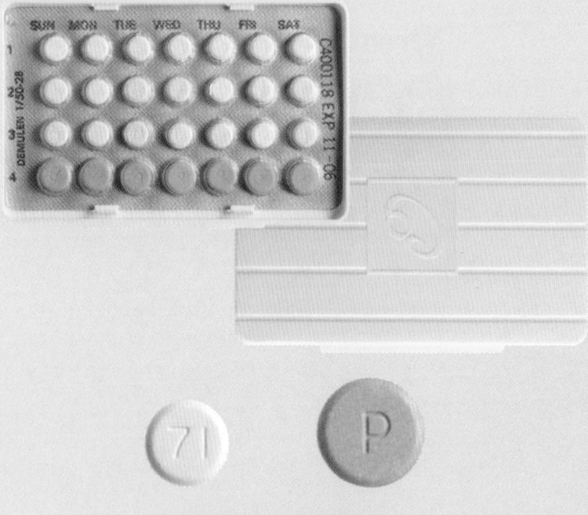

Demulen® 1/50
(ethinyl estradiol/ethynodiol diacetate)

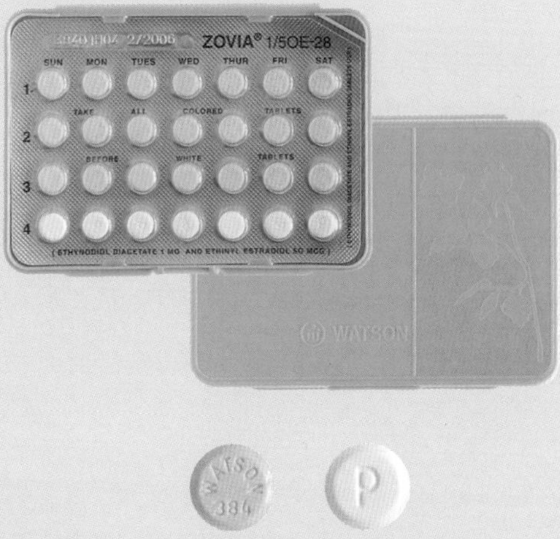

Zovia® 1/50E
(ethinyl estradiol/ethynodiol diacetate)

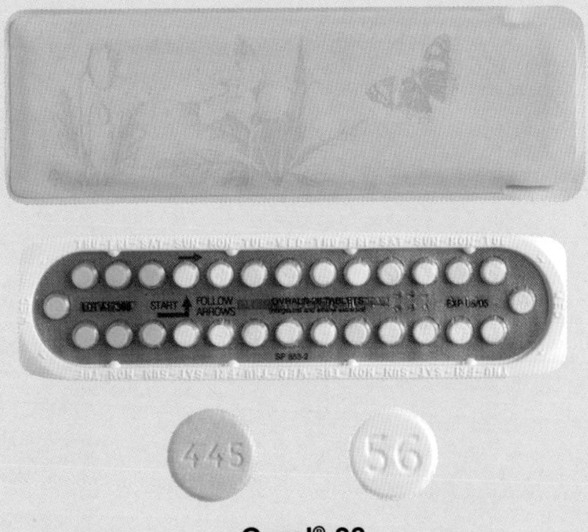

Ovral®-28
(ethinyl estradiol/norgestrel)

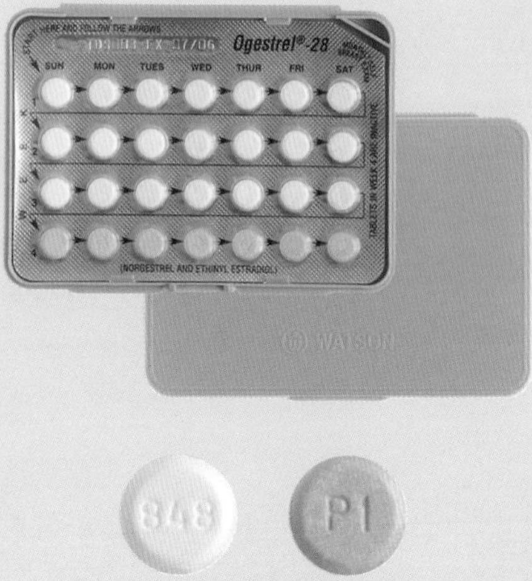

Ogestrel®
(ethinyl estradiol/norgestrel)

Section B: Multiphasic

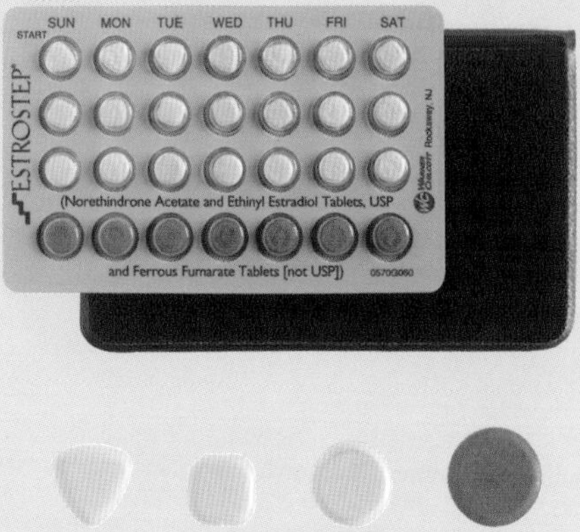

Estrostep® Fe
(ethinyl estradiol/norethindrone acetate)

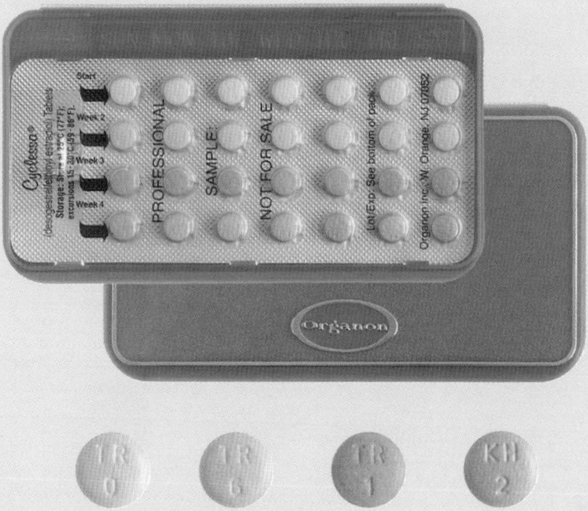

Cyclessa®
(ethinyl estradiol/desogestrel)

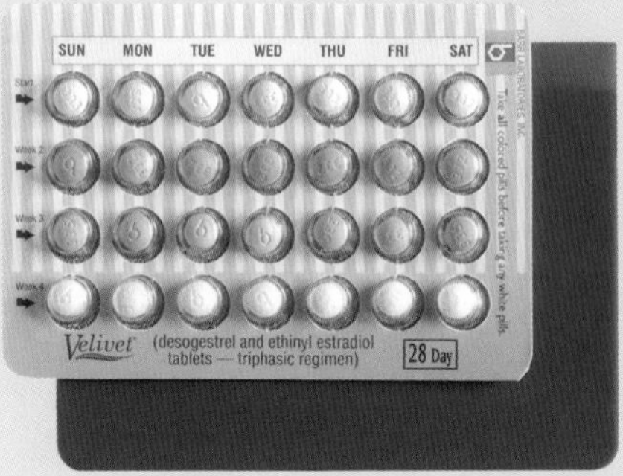

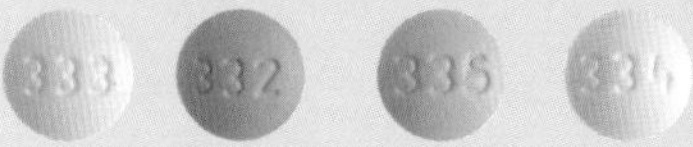

Velivet™
(ethinyl estradiol/desogestrel)

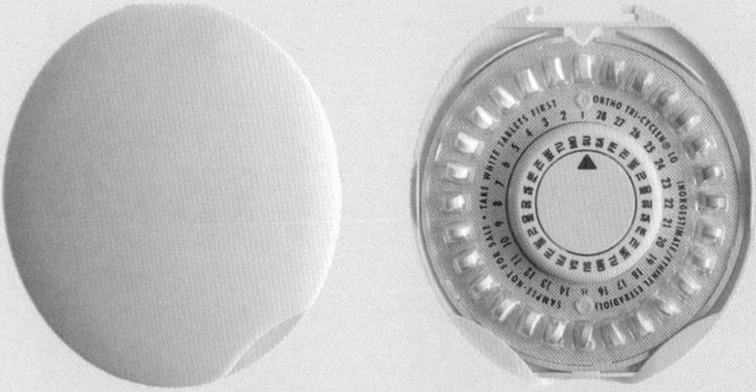

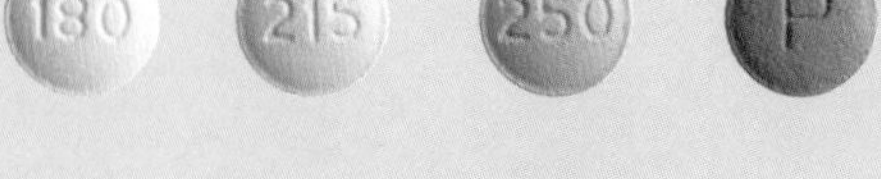

Ortho Tri-Cyclen® Lo
(ethinyl estradiol/norgestimate)

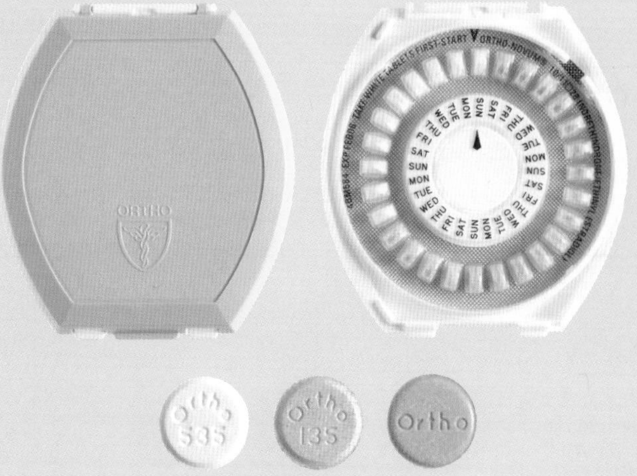

Ortho-Novum® 10/11
(ethinyl estradiol/norethindrone)

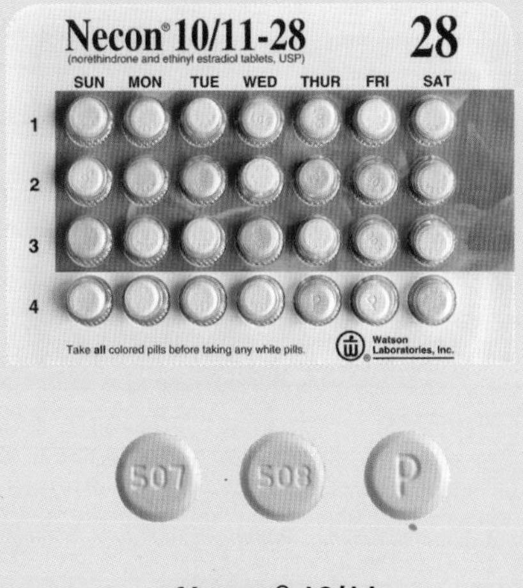

Necon® 10/11-28
28
(norethindrone and ethinyl estradiol tablets, USP)
SUN MON TUE WED THUR FRI SAT
1
2
3
4
Take all colored pills before taking any white pills.
Watson Laboratories, Inc.
507
508
P

Necon® 10/11
(ethinyl estradiol/norethindrone)

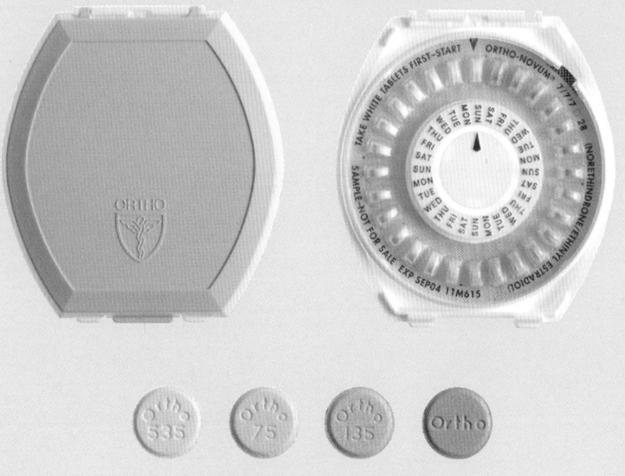

Ortho-Novum® 7/7/7
(ethinyl estradiol/norethindrone)

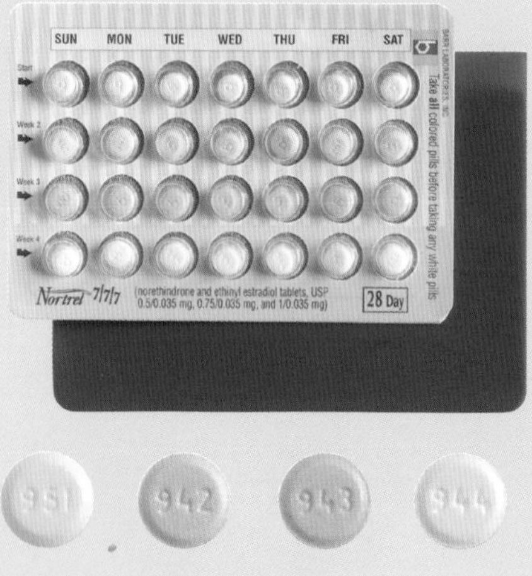

Nortrel® 7/7/7
(ethinyl estradiol/norethindrone)

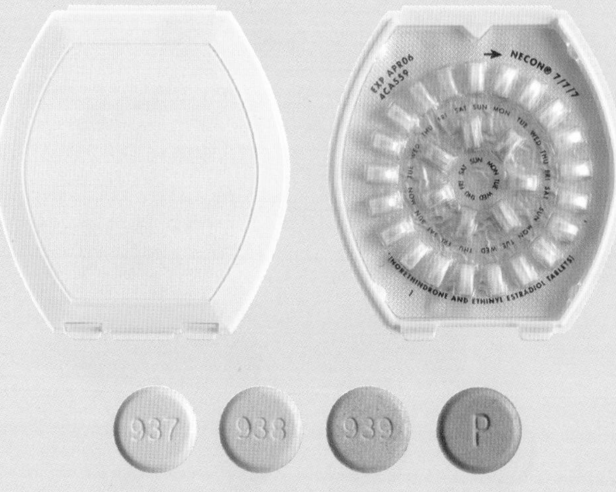

Necon® 7/7/7
(ethinyl estradiol/norethindrone)

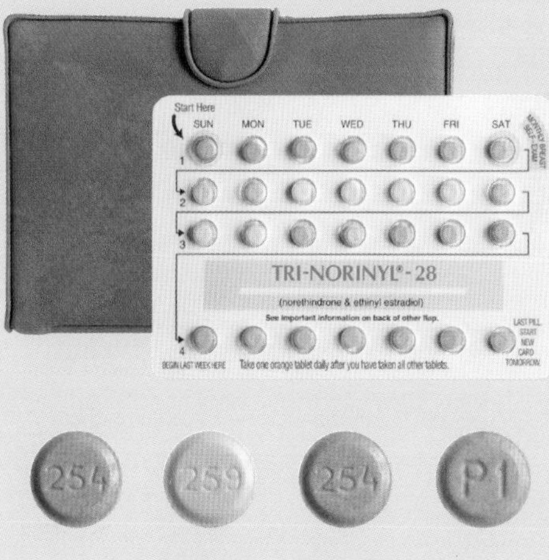

Tri-Norinyl®-28
(ethinyl estradiol/norethindrone)

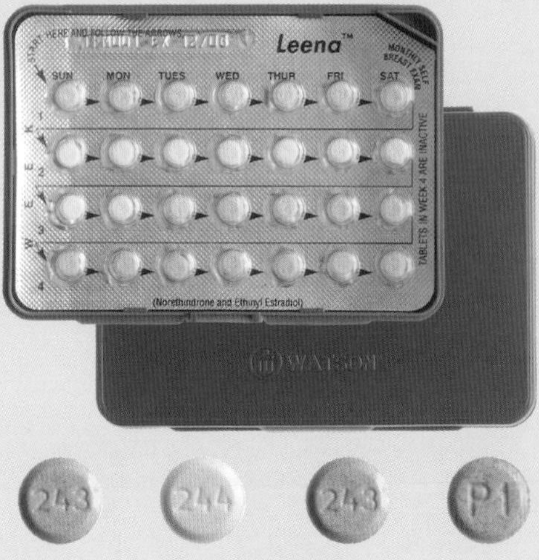

Leena™
(ethinyl estradiol/norethindrone)

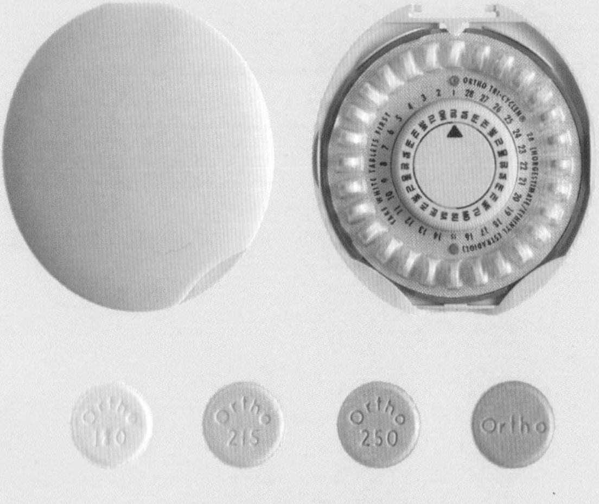

Ortho Tri-Cyclen®
(ethinyl estradiol/norgestimate)

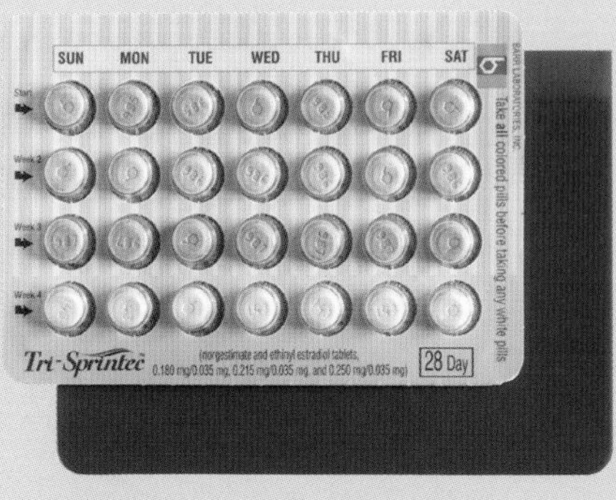

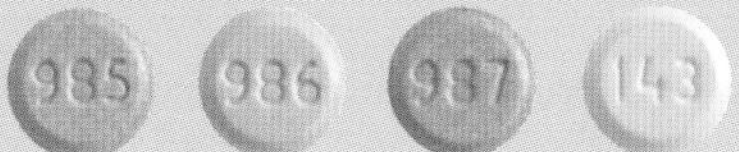

Tri-Sprintec®

(ethinyl estradiol/norgestimate)

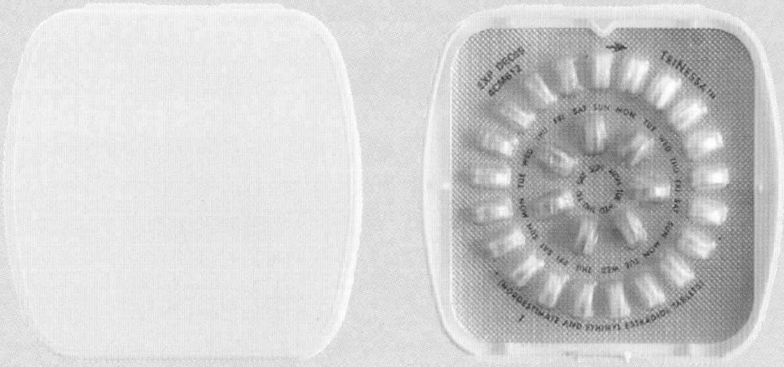

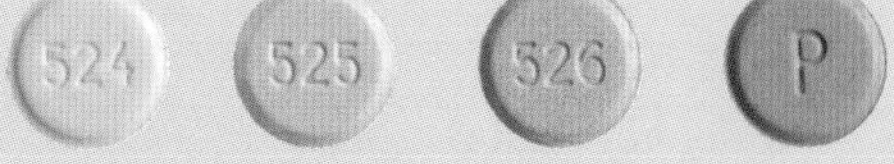

TriNessa®

(ethinyl estradiol/norgestimate)

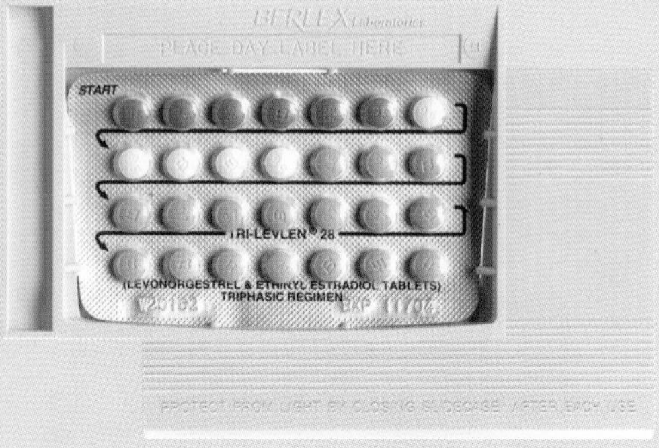

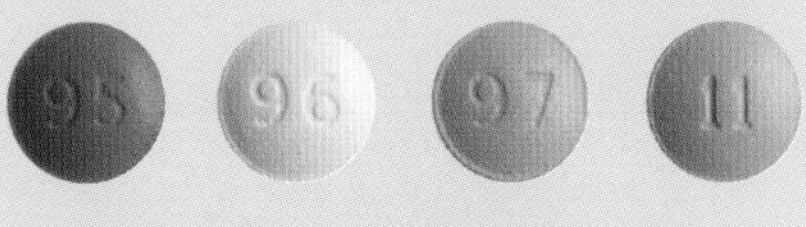

Tri-Levlen® 28
(ethinyl estradiol/levonorgestrel)

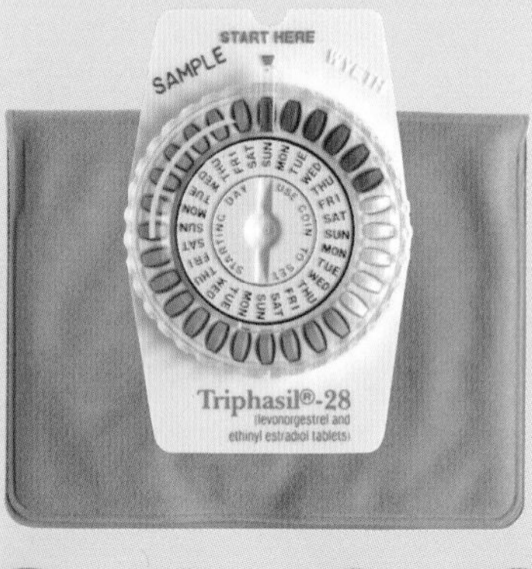

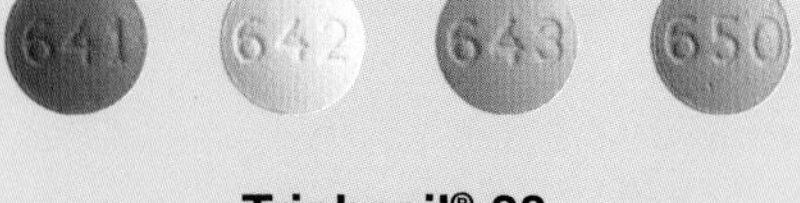

Triphasil®-28
(ethinyl estradiol/levonorgestrel)